THE STENGLER
CANCER-REVERSING
PROTOCOL

Your personal guide to the
most powerful natural cancer therapies

Table of Contents

How to Live Longer... and Better... With the Incredible Cancer-Fighting Power of Ascorbate Therapy

"Significant advances rarely came from within orthodox medicine... most were made by mavericks."[1] This statement—spoken by a true pioneer in the use of ascorbate therapy, also known as intravenous vitamin C, for people with cancer...Hugh Riordan MD—is as true today as when it was first uttered. And there's no area of medicine that conventional medicine, and the pharmaceutical companies, have more of a stranglehold on accepted standards of medical therapy than the disease of cancer.

Surgery, chemotherapy, and radiation are the standard treatments when it comes to cancer. Sometimes they're even beneficial. But they often come with brutal side effects, a poor track record for long-term survival, and a quality of life you wouldn't wish on your own worst enemy.

Now, after decades of disappointing results and horrendous side effects, the American public has started to realize that there are alternatives, and more and more people are seeking Integrative Cancer Care. Doctors like me are incorporating a variety of nutritional and holistic therapies to improve patient outcomes and provide better quality of life for people with cancer. Intravenous vitamin C is proving to be one of the best all around Integrative Therapies.

The conventional medicine viewpoint has always been that cancer can't be treated with holistic therapies. Tell that to the Chinese, Japanese, German and Swiss doctors who have been taking an integrative approach to cancer for decades now. By combining the best of conventional and natural healing methods—or in some cases natural therapies alone—they're achieving better results with significantly less side effects than standard conventional care alone. Yet here in America, in the not-so-distant past, doctors have lost their licenses or have even been prosecuted by the U.S. government for choosing to use humane integrative treatments with their own patients.

Holistic therapies save lives!

Case in point, Stanislaw R. Burzynski, M.D., Ph.D developed a breakthrough treatment in which patients are given antineoplastons, peptides and amino acids taken from the human body that activate cancer-fighting genes. Even though Dr. Burzynki had great success with this treatment as demonstrated in clinical trials and confirmed patient cases (including patients who had terminal or difficult-to-treat cancers) he was attacked by the medical establishment for over a decade because his treatments were not FDA approved.

The good news is that an increasing number of doctors, including oncologists, are opening up to the idea of Integrative Oncology Therapy. It not only makes rational sense to support the body's immune system and help the body to detoxify from conventional treatments, but also to use natural therapies shown to have direct anti-cancer effects.

Recently I attended a three-day conference with leading integrative doctors including oncologists. Most of the presentations focused on the use of intravenous therapies (substances given directly into the vein of a patient to bypass their digestive tract so higher, therapeutic doses can be used). The research provided was nothing short of astounding.

For years holistic doctors have noted the positive effects of nutritional intravenous therapies such as vitamin C on their patients. I myself have personally witnessed patients having better outcomes in terms of length and quality of life. However, little *published* data has existed to present to the medical world. Studies, especially good ones, require a lot of money to fund. But pharmaceutical companies, which by far have the deepest pockets when it comes to funding research, don't have an interest in paying for such studies since natural substances can't be patented and will not generate huge stacks of cash.

But things are looking up and the tide is turning. Some high-quality studies have been completed, and many more are on their way. Much of the research presented at this three-day conference was on the exciting field of Intravenous Vitamin C (IVC) and I want to share some of it with you here. But first, let's take a quick look at the history of IVC.

Tens of thousands have already been helped with IV vitamin C

The most famous proponent of vitamin C was Linus Pauling (1901-1994), a molecular biologist and the only person to ever win two unshared Nobel Prizes. Most agree he was one of the two most influential scientists of the 20th century.

Pauling published over 1000 books and articles, most on scientific subjects. He coined the term "orthomolecular" which means the "right molecules in the right concentration." Orthomolecular medicine focuses on using natural substances such as nutrients like vitamin C to restore the optimum environment of the body by correcting imbalances or deficiencies. In orthomolecular medicine we often use doses much higher than what's currently recommended by the conventional establishment.

Pauling, along with Dr. Ewan Cameron, former Chief of Surgery at Vale of Leven Hospital in Scotland, published research in the 1970s demonstrating that IVC at a dose of usually 10 grams daily for 10 days, followed by daily doses of 10 grams orally in terminal cancer patients, led to an astounding 4-fold increase in life expectancy.[2] Of course 10 grams of IVC is a fraction of the 50 to 100 grams that's typically used for people with cancer today.

In 1979 Cameron and Pauling published their book, *Cancer and Vitamin C*, which described their clinical experience with vitamin C and cancer. What happened next was devastating. Researchers at Mayo Clinic conducted two studies using 10 grams daily of <u>oral</u> vitamin C in late-stage cancer patients. They never received Intravenous Vitamin C as the research by Cameron and Pauling indicated was needed. Their conclusion was that vitamin C had no statistical benefit.[3] Linus Pauling diligently wrote rebuttal letters pointing out that the Mayo studies did **not** replicate his and Cameron's research. Unfortunately, the medical community took the Mayo studies as conclusive evidence against the benefits of IVC and it has been shunned by conventional medicine until this day.

I mentioned Dr. Hugh Riordan earlier. He's no longer alive, but his work continues on through the Riordan Clinic in Wichita, Kansas, which has used IVC to help tens of thousands of cancer patients. The research arm of the clinic has been conducting and publishing research on vitamin C for the past 15 years.

Dr. Riordan's RECNAC (cancer spelled backwards) research team has published 20 papers on vitamin C and cancer. According to the clinic, "RECNAC data has shown that vitamin C is toxic to tumor cells without sacrificing the performance of chemotherapy."[4] In fact, the team has found that not only is IVC effective, it's safe as well. Similar to my experiences with IVC, they state, "There have been no serious complications. The most common adverse events reported were nausea, edema, and dry mouth or skin; and these were generally minor."[5] You can read about their research at www.riordanclinic.org.

Kick your immune response into high gear with IVC

When you administer vitamin C intravenously, blood levels of the vitamin can reach levels 70 to 100 times higher than oral vitamin C. This is important because oral vitamin C generally can't reach high enough blood levels to effectively kill cancer cells. Research by the Riordan Clinic has found that tumor cells become susceptible to high dose IVC at plasma levels of 350 to 400 mg/dL.[6]

Your immune system naturally produces some hydrogen peroxide in response to infections and cancer. High doses of IVC kick this natural process into high gear. Hydrogen peroxide acts as an oxidant, helping to destroy cancer and other foreign invaders. IVC augments what your immune system is already doing, making the process much more effective.

Normal healthy cells are able to neutralize the effects of hydrogen peroxide with an enzyme known as catalase. Since cancer cells lack this enzyme it leads to cell death. A study in the *Proceedings of the National Academy of Science of the United States of America* showed that IVC selectively kills cancer cells by delivering hydrogen peroxide to tissues.[7]

High dose IVC also acts as an antioxidant, but this action appears to be a bit less powerful than its oxidant effect. As an antioxidant, however, vitamin C helps to control the inflammation that stokes the fires of cancer cell replication. While many conventional doctors are concerned about the antioxidant effect of vitamin C for patients undergoing chemotherapy and radiation (which produce a lot of oxidants), this concern seems largely unfounded in light of recent research. In addition, Naturopathic Doctor Paul Anderson has done extensive research on published interactions between vitamin C and common chemotherapy medications and other common cancer drugs. His research finds little in the way of negative interactions.[8]

As Dr. Hunninghake from the Riordan Clinic has pointed out, conventional therapies such as certain chemotherapies and radiation work by increasing oxidation and inducing cancer cell death (apoptosis). However, they *also* damage the control mechanisms for cell death including the p53 gene which suppresses tumor formation. This allows therapy-resistant cells to thrive, while leaving your other cells with less control over cancer formation at the same time. He notes that IVC acts as an oxidative treatment helping to destroy cancer cells, while the gentle antioxidant effects of the vitamin protect and repair the cells so they have control over cell replication such as the p53 gene.[9]

Douse inflammation and lower your CRP levels

Inflammation plays an important role in cancer formation and promotes the replication of cancer cells, their survival, and their migration throughout the body. One of the traditional blood tests for monitoring inflammation in the body is C reactive protein (CRP).

In one study of over 274,000 people, about one third of deaths in a community were due to cancer. Those with an increased CRP had a higher risk of dying from cancer than from any other cause including cardiovascular disease.[10]

Research also shows that your level of CRP is a good predictor of cancer survival.[11] Research at the Riordan Clinic has found that a series of IVC sessions can lower CRP by approximately 75%. They concluded that this reduction in CRP correlated with a drop in tumor markers including the PSA in prostate cancer.[12]

High dose IVC also aids in detoxification and improving cell energy function. More specifically it improves oxygenation of the cells. Cancer cells don't do well in an oxygenated environment and IVC shifts cells to an aerobic (utilizing oxygen) environment instead of the anaerobic (without oxygen) state that leads to the creation of more cells.

According to Hunninghake, his research team has documented seven ways that IVC fights cancer. Hunninghake's Seven Hallmarks of Cancer that IVC deals with are:[13]

1. Self-sufficiency of growth signals
2. Insensitivity to antigrowth signals
3. Evasion of apoptosis (cell death)
4. Unlimited proliferation potential
5. Enhanced angiogenesis (blood-vessel supply to the tumor)
6. Tissue invasion and metastasis
7. Inflammatory microenvironment

IVC therapy is extending lives... yours could be next

One of the leading research institutions for studying the effects of IVC in people with cancer is the Bastyr University Integrative Oncology Research Center (BIORC), in Seattle. The Center opened in 2009, after receiving a grant from a man whose wife had died from breast cancer who wanted research to be done to find out if there was a better way to treat the disease. Since then, 521 cancer patients have been enrolled in a

New Study Confirms the Natural Cancer-Killing Power of Vitamin C

Vitamin C has been underrated by conventional medicine for treating cancer patients for decades.

Well, the cat's out of the bag now as a major new study of the benefits of vitamin C confirms that a powerful therapy used for decades in natural medicine can kill cancer cells without doing a drop of damage to normal cells.

It's plain old vitamin C.

In high enough levels, vitamin C causes the production of hydrogen peroxide in the blood, and hydrogen peroxide is like kryptonite to cancer cells. As a result, the C was able to wipe out both human and animal ovarian cancer cells when delivered alongside chemo in the new study.

That's a lab-dish experiment. But the study didn't stop there.

In a follow-up experiment on 27 human patients with stage III and IV ovarian cancer, vitamin C was shown to boost the cancer-fighting powers of chemo while limiting its toxic side effects.

In fact, the patients given vitamin C suffered almost no side effects at all, according to the study of the benefits of vitamin C in the journal *Science Translational Medicine*.

Amazing, right? Not really, actually, because this isn't exactly new.

We've known about the cancer-fighting powers of vitamin C for decades.

What's really amazing is how effective Big Pharma and its government pals have been at hiding this from the public — and they've been doing it in one of the most underhanded ways imaginable.

Back in the 1970s, a major mainstream study supposedly proved that vitamin C does nothing to fight cancer. But the study was designed to fail, testing only oral supplements instead of the high intravenous doses we know are so effective.

Ever since that little bait-and-switch, they've claimed research "proves" that C doesn't work against cancer, using the study to persecute (and even prosecute) any doctor heroic enough to offer this life-saving treatment.

The new study turns the tables, because this one finally used intravenous C instead of oral supplements — and the results speak for themselves.

The reason for the big difference between oral and intravenous is something you can actually see — something you almost certainly have seen if you've ever taken a vitamin C supplement and noticed your pee turn bright yellow afterward.

That happens because oral C passes through you very quickly. While your body can still use some of it as it flows through, it can never build up in the high levels needed to create the hydrogen peroxide I mentioned earlier.

Intravenous C can, as the new study shows quite clearly.

In this case, it was delivered alongside chemo. But in reality, I've found it can actually be used in place of chemo in many cases.

Whether or not you need chemo is a decision I'll leave up to you and your doctor. Either way, make sure the benefits of vitamin C are part of your treatment — and don't stop there.

Other nutrients that can help make cancer treatments more effective and less toxic when delivered intravenously include B vitamins, amino acids, glutathione and zinc.

study series involving all stages of the disease. Originally patients were only from the Seattle area, but as word spread cancer patients from all over the country have come to the clinic to participate in the research.

The most common types of cancers seen at BIORC are breast, lung, colon, pancreatic, and brain cancers, as well as Merkel cell carcinoma (a type of skin cancer). Approximately 30% of the patients seen at the clinic have been in stage IV or the end stage of the disease where the cancer has spread. They are treated with nutritional therapies and Intravenous Vitamin C and other holistic intravenous therapies.

Leanna Standish, PhD, ND, Lac, from the School of Public Health at the University of Washington and BIORC has been the lead investigator in analyzing the data coming from the center. She's been comparing the data to The Seattle Cancer Care Alliance, a world renowned conventional cancer treatment center in the same area. While the research is ongoing, the data the clinic has gathered so far has been spectacular.[14,15]

For example:

- **Eight patients with stage IV colon cancer**—Three years after their care at the clinic began, 80% were still alive; only 15% of Seattle Cancer Care patients in a similar group were alive at three years.

- **Twelve consecutive patients with stage IV lung cancer**—After being treated at BIORC, 64% were still alive at three years. The Seattle Cancer Care reports a 15% survival rate at three years and SEER (National Statistics) show just a 3% survival rate.

- **Eleven consecutive stage III ovarian cancer patients**—At three years, 83% of them are still alive. The SEER national data reports a 49% survival rate at three years.

- **Forty six stage IV breast cancer patients**—The eighteen of the 46 that received IVC therapy had a 31.1% survival rate at five years compared to just 22.2% for those who had not received IV therapy.

IVC can also be used at lower doses to enhance the quality of life for people with cancer (and other diseases). Two published studies have demonstrated this benefit. One found that IV vitamin C significantly reduced side effects caused by the cancer, chemotherapy, or radiation including nausea, loss of appetite, fatigue, depression, sleep disorders, dizziness and bleeding. No side effects were documented.[16]

Another very recent study involved a clinical trial of 25 women with ovarian cancer. Thirteen of the women received chemotherapy and vitamin C by IV. Researchers found that those volunteers who received IVC were less likely to report side effects from the chemotherapy than those who received chemotherapy alone. The same researchers also found that IVC promoted cell death in ovarian cells grown in culture.[17] Another study found patients reported significantly less fatigue, nausea/vomiting, pain, and appetite loss after receiving IVC.[18]

Getting down to details on IVC therapy

A dosage of IVC usually ranges between 25 to 75 grams. This is because the desired oxidative effect typically takes place at around 25 grams or higher. But, depending on the person, the optimal oxidative dosage may vary. A patient will normally be given a lower amount, such as 20 grams, to start and with subsequent IV's the level is increased.

IVC formulas normally only contain minerals to balance blood electrolytes such as magnesium, calcium and potassium. Sodium bicarbonate is also added to neutralize the acidity of the solution to prevent any possible vein irritation.

Research by Dr. Anderson has found that it takes a minimum of 12 to 15 treatments to assess whether or not the therapy will work for someone. Patients usually get one to three treatments per week, and each treatment takes about an hour and a half to two hours.

I've found that side effects are uncommon. However, it's important for the patient to eat a well-balanced meal before the treatment and to drink plenty water before, during, and after the treatment. IVC can lower blood sugar levels and be mildly dehydrating. There's the possibility that blood calcium and potassium levels can be lowered with the treatment. This is prevented by including them in the IVC solution. Vein irritation and pain can occasionally occur, but this is normally prevented or resolved by increasing the amount of sodium bicarbonate in the IVC solution and slowing the drip rate. If you have a port (a medical appliance that's surgically placed under the skin to give access to a vein) then vein irritation is rare.

Your doctor should analyze your lab work, including blood and urine testing, before starting IVC and should run tests again periodically during your treatments. If you have decreased kidney filtration or liver disease you will need to be monitored more closely, although problems from IVC for those with these conditions are still rare. You should also have a marker known as G6PD tested *before* starting high dose IVC. This is an inherited condition known as Glucose 6 Phosphate Dehydrogenase. If you have the marker your cells can't tolerate high dose vitamin C. It is more common in people of African, Asian, Middle Eastern, and Mediterranean descent.

If you know of someone who has cancer then be sure to let them know about the benefit of IVC. We administer a lot of high dose IVC at my clinic to people with a variety of cancers and have seen a lot of success. Good resources for finding a doctor close to you include American College for Advancement in Medicine (ACAM) at www.acam.org, Bastyr Integrative Oncology Research Center (BIORC) at www.bastyr.edu, Anderson Medical Specialty Associates (in the Seattle area) www.amsa1.com, and the Riordan Clinic at www.riordanclinic.org.

Article Citations

1. Hunninghake, Ron. Adjunctive IVC Therapy Help Cancer Patients Update. 3rd Annual Conference and Expo IV Therapies 2014. Integrative Oncology. January 25, 2014.

2. Cameron E, Campbell A. The orthomolecular treatment of cancer II. Clinical trial of high-dose ascorbic acid supplements in advanced human cancer. Chem Biol Interact. 1974;9:285–315.

3. Creagan ET, Moertel CG, O'Fallon JR, et al: Failure of high-dose vitamin C (ascorbic acid) therapy to benefit patients with advanced cancer. N Engl J Med, 1979; 301: 687-690.

4. Riordan Clinic.org website. Accessed February 22, 2014 at www.riordanclinic.org/research/research-studies/vitaminc/

5. Ibid, www.riordanclinic.org/research/research-studies/vitaminc/tumor/

6. Hunninghake, Ron. Adjunctive IVC Therapy Help Cancer Patients Update. 3rd Annual Conference and Expo IV Therapies 2014 Integrative Oncology. January 25, 2014.

7. Chen Q1, Espey MG, Krishna MC, Mitchell JB, Corpe CP, Buettner GR, Shacter E, Levine M. Pharmacologic ascorbic acid concentrations selectively kill cancer cells: action as a pro-drug to deliver hydrogen peroxide to tissues. Proc Natl Acad Sci U S A. 2005 Sep 20;102(38):13604-9. Epub, September 12, 2005.

8. Anderson, Paul. Updated Data Review and Policies for concurrent use at Anderson Medical Specialty Associates, Southwest College of Naturopathic Medicine Research Institute and Medical Center and Bastyr University Clinical Research Center. 3rd Annual Conference and Expo IV Therapies 2014. Integrative Oncology. January 25, 2014.

9. Hunninghake, Ron. Ibid.

10. Marsik C, Kazemi-Shirazi L, Schickbauer T, Winkler S, Joukhadar C, Wagner OF, Endler G. C-reactive protein and all-cause mortality in a large hospital-based cohort. Clin Chem. 2008 Feb;54(2):343-9.

11. Mahmoud FA, Rivera NI. The role of C-reactive protein as a prognostic indicator in advanced cancer. Current Oncology Report 2002;4:250–5.

12. Riordan Clinic. Org website, ibid.

13. Hunninghake, Ron. Ibid.

14. Medscape.com. Can Integrative Oncology Extend Life in Advanced Disease? Accessed February 23, 2014 at www.medscape.com/viewarticle/813217

15. Anderson, Paul. Updated Data Review and Policies for Concurrent Use at Anderson Medical Specialty Associates, Southwest College of Naturopathic Medicine Research Institute and Medical Center and Bastyr University Clinical Research Center. 3rd Annual Conference and Expo IV Therapies 2014. Integrative Oncology. January 25, 2014.

16. Vollbracht, C. et al., 2011. Intravenous vitamin C administration improves quality of life in breast cancer patients during chemo-radiotherapy and aftercare: results of a retrospective, multicentre, epidemiological cohort study in Germany. In Vivo. Volume 82, pp. 983-90.

17. Nature.com. Vitamin C injections ease ovarian-cancer treatments. Accessed February 23, 2014 at http://www.nature.com/news/vitamin-c-injections-ease-ovarian-cancer-treatments-1.14673

18. Yeom, C., Jung, G. & Song, K., 2007. Changes of terminal cancer patient's health related quality of life after high dose vitamin C administration. Korean Medical Science Volume 22, pp. 7-11.

CHAPTER 2

Dr. Stengler's Ultimate Cancer-Fighting Diet

Supercharge Your Immune System and Fight Cancer with the Secret "Cloud Mushroom" Remedy from the East

Have you ever heard of turkey tail? No, I'm not talking about the tail feathers of our favorite thanksgiving bird. It's actually a mushroom with a rather colorful name and a surprising ability.

The turkey tail is a potent medicinal mushroom that has been found to boost your immune system. In fact, there are over 400 published studies showing just how powerful this mushroom is. Several human studies have even shown that it may be able to fight cancer. But don't feel bad if you haven't heard of turkey tail before, because even most cancer doctors are clueless about this "secret" wonder of nature.

The truth is, most mainstream <u>doctors</u> don't even know medicinal mushrooms like turkey tail exist. Not so surprising since drug companies sponsor both the medical schools they attend and the continuing education seminars they go to. And, of course, drug companies have no interest in cheap natural remedies that they can't patent. Individual doctors can, of course, venture a look outside of the box and do their own research, but the reality is most don't.

Even worse, doctors are often so brainwashed that they develop a bias against natural therapies. They're not willing to admit that some natural remedies work even if the science <u>proves</u> that they do. I've seen this happen countless times with my own patients who respond well to a complementary therapy I recommend. Their oncologists often ignore the positive results. Or, if they do acknowledge them, they refuse to learn more about the therapy that led to them.

Talking turkey tail mushrooms

Although here in the West few of us have ever heard of turkey tail, it's well known in East Asian medicine. In fact, in Japan and China, there's a long history of using it in both traditional and modern medical practices. In traditional Chinese medicine the mushroom is used to treat pulmonary infections, hepatitis, and cancer. And in Japan it's a folk remedy commonly used to treat cancer.

One mushroom, many uses

In Japan and China, turkey tail extract is commonly used for immune enhancement for those who have had surgery, are undergoing chemotherapy, or are receiving radiation treatments.

The scientific names for turkey tail mushrooms are Coriolus versicolor and Trametes versicolor. The Latin translation of Trametes is "one who is thin" and versicolor means "variously colored."

The fungus grows naturally on dead logs and on trees around the world. It has a fan-shaped, multicolored cap that some say resembles the tail feathers of a turkey. However, in Japan you would ask for *kawaratake* or "the mushroom by the river bank." And in China you'd look for *yun zhi* or the "cloud mushroom."

In the 1960s a Japanese scientist saw that a neighbor with late stage stomach cancer was treating himself with turkey tail. He became interested in the mushroom and he and his colleagues began to study it. Eventually the group developed an extract that they named PSK, an abbreviation for polysaccharide-K. Soon after, Chinese researchers developed their own version of the extract naming it PSP, an abbreviation for polysaccharide-peptide. Here in America, non-drug versions of turkey tail extract are available in the form of a nutritional supplement.

Building "super immunities" with glucans

The secret to the immune boosting power of many mushrooms are compounds called glucans. Turkey tail has its own unique "super" version of glucans. These glucans are pulled from the mushrooms using a special water extraction process. The result is a powerful immune enhancing extract.

Research shows that these special glucans pass right through the gut wall and into the bloodstream unchanged. (This means that when they go to work they're just as potent as when they were extracted.) Next, the extract switches on receptors on your immune cells, including neutrophils, monocytes/ macrophages, natural killer cells, and T- and B-lymphocytes. So, in other words, the glucans essentially supercharge your entire immune system not only turning on your body's own cancer killers, but also the immune cells that fight off bacteria and viruses.

The infection connection

Turkey tail mushrooms are great immune builders. They can be used to help treat infections of the respiratory tract and for chronic viral infections such as hepatitis B.

Turkey tail is obviously great for building up your immune system. But what I prescribe it for most often is as a complimentary therapy for treating cancer. Studies show it does the most good for: esophageal, lung, colon, and stomach cancers.

Leaving lung cancer behind

One ten-year study looked at how good turkey tail extract (PSK) is at protecting your health when you're *already* ill. Researchers recruited 185 people with lung cancer who were getting radiation. Half of the group received a placebo and the other half received the PSK extract. And it turns out that the mushroom does an excellent job of protecting the immune system of lung cancer patients.

The researchers found that those receiving the turkey tail did much better overall than those on the placebo. The 5-year survival rates of the patients who got the extract were 39 percent for those who had stage I or stage II cancers, and 22 percent for those who had stage III. And while those numbers may not seem huge at first glance, when you compare them to the placebo group's numbers of 16 percent and 5 percent it's instantly clear just how significant a difference the extract made.

Plus, those lung cancer patients who were 70 years old or older who got the PSK had a much better chance of surviving than those that only got radiation.

Conquering colon cancer

Another ten-year study showed just how good turkey tail is against colon cancer. The randomized double-blind trial divided a group of 111 volunteers with colon cancer into two. After surgery for colorectal cancer the first group of 56 patients took a turkey tail extract (PSK). The second group of 55 was given a placebo.

The results were pretty stunning. The rate of patients in remission (or disease-free) in the PSK group was <u>more than double</u> that of the placebo group! Researchers also found that the PSK patient's white blood cells showed, in their words, "remarkable enhancement in their activities." (White blood cells are the ones that fight disease by attacking things that don't belong in the body like germs, bacteria, and cancers. So anything that boosts their abilities is welcome in the fight against cancer.)

Striking back at stomach cancer

Turkey tail may be an important player in the fight against stomach cancer. One study, published in *The Lancet*, examined the effect of PSK in stomach cancer patients. All of the volunteers had stomach surgery and were starting chemotherapy. The two hundred sixty-two patients got either standard treatment alone or with PSK.

The survival rate of the group using both turkey tail extract and chemotherapy was 73 percent after 5 years. The group who got chemotherapy alone had a survival rate of only 60 percent. The researchers said that PSK had "a restorative effect in patients who had been immunosuppressed by both recent surgery and subsequent chemotherapy."

Slashing chemo and radiation side effects

One of the biggest sins in medicine today is that <u>proven</u> complementary therapies are being ignored and aren't being used on cancer patients. The fact is, turkey tail can work wonders when it comes to beating the toxic side effects of cancer treatments.

Researchers at the University of Shanghai, wanted to find out if Coriolus polysaccharides (PSP) could reduce the side effects of chemotherapy or radiation. They recruited 650 people with cancer who were undergoing chemotherapy and radiation and gave them either PSP or a placebo. Then they measured how severe the side effects from the cancer treatments were in both groups. It turns out that those volunteers who received PSP had a lot fewer side effects than those that got the placebo.

And as any one who has been through the nightmare of chemo or radiation can tell you, the cure can sometimes seem worse than the disease. So fewer side effects are a Godsend.

Talk to your doc about turkey tail

If you have esophageal, lung, stomach, or colon cancer I recommend you talk to your oncologist about turkey tail. Now don't be surprised if you meet some resistance at first. But remember, the science proves that the mushroom extract can reduce the side effects of conventional therapies, supercharge your cancer killing cells, and even reduce your chances of a cancer coming back. So if your doctor is willing to take an honest look at the evidence he should also be willing to give it a try.

And if after looking at all the studies he's still resisting it might be time for you to find a new doctor. Your life could *literally* depend on it.

I usually recommend 1,000 to 1,500 mg of a standard hot water extract twice a day (of course make sure to check with your *own* doctor before starting supplementation). As with any immune modulator you should not use turkey tail extract if you've had an organ transplant, or if you're taking immunosuppressive drugs. Side effects from turkey tail supplements are rare. Look for a standardized extract at your local health food store or from your holistic doctor.

Citations:

1. Hayakawa K, Mitsuhashi N, Saito Y, Takahashi M, Katano S, Shiojima K, Furuta M, Niibe H. Effect of krestin (PSK) as adjuvant treatment on the prognosis after radical radiotherapy in patients with non-small cell lung cancer. Anticancer Res. 1993 Sep-Oct;13(5C):1815-20.

2. Torisu M, Hayashi Y, Ishimitsu T, Fujimura T, Iwasaki K, Katano M, Yamamoto H, Kimura Y, Takesue M, et al. Significant prolongation of disease-free period gained by oral polysaccharide K (PSK) administration after curative surgical operation of colorectal cancer. Cancer Immunol Immunother. 1990;31(5):261-8.

3. Nakazato H, Koike A, Saji S, Ogawa N, Sakamoto J. Efficacy of immunochemotherapy as adjuvant treatment after curative resection of gastric cancer. Study Group of Immunochemotherapy with PSK for Gastric Cancer. Lancet. 1994 May 7;343(8906):1122-6.

4. Sun Z et al. The ameliorative effect of PSP on the toxic and side reaction of chemo and radiotherapy of cancers. In: Yang O, ed. Advanced Research in PSP. Hong Kong: Hong Kong Association for Health Care Ltd; 1999.

High Protein Foods
Can Boost Cancer Risk

Our diet is killing you.

That cheeseburger may be the death of you — and I'm not kidding.

Too much meat, cheese and other unhealthy high protein foods in middle age can quadruple your risk of death from cancer, according to a major new study.

That makes a Dairy Queen habit as bad for your health as smoking, and the risks don't end with cancer.

If you get 20 percent of your diet from animal protein and high protein foods, you could also face four times the risk of death from diabetes and double the risk of an early death from any cause, according to the new study in *Cell Metabolism*.

Cutting protein in your diet down to 10 percent or less, on the other hand, will cut your risk death from any cause in half and death from cancer by 25 percent.

Surprised? Don't be.

Part of the reason is likely in your hormones, specifically a hormone known as insulin growth factor-1, or IGF-1.

When you're young and growing, you need plenty of it. But as you get older, you need less. In fact, as you get older, too much IGF-1 can hurt you.

This shouldn't be a problem because of the ingenious way in which we've been designed: Your body naturally produces plenty of IGF-1 when you are young and need the stuff, and much less as you age.

But bad habits can disrupt this natural process, especially the bad habits of the modern junk-food diet, which can cause your IGF-1 factory to start pumping out hormones overtime just when production should be tailing off.

Of course, that's one reason — but I don't believe it's the only reason.

Not all high protein foods are unhealthy, but people who eat the most animal proteins tend to be people who aren't making healthy choices. They're eating cheeseburgers and drinking milkshakes.

Eat quality proteins such as fish, lean meats and poultry, and I'm sure crossing the 10 percent threshold won't hurt you.

If there's one upside to the study, it's that it also finds that higher levels of protein can actually help extend lives in seniors.

This may be in part because seniors are so low in IGF-1 that even a bump in production from protein won't hurt. And it may also be because seniors tend to lose muscle mass as they age and a diet too low in protein can accelerate that process.

Loss of muscle leads to weakness, loss of balance, falls, breaks, loss of independence and a higher risk of an early death.

Healthy proteins (and amino acids) can support your muscle so you stay strong.

In other words, don't celebrate your 65th birthday under the Golden Arches. Instead, continue to make sure your proteins are quality proteins, and limit your red meat intake.

For a balanced diet with just the right amount of healthy proteins at every age, I recommend a Mediterranean lifestyle rich in lean meats, fatty fish, olive oil, nuts, seeds and all the fresh produce you care to enjoy.

This diet has been proven to cut the risk of cancer and diabetes. (Yes, precisely the diseases that a diet too high in protein can cause.)

Fight Cancer Fatigue and Beat Exhaustion with this Native American Herbal Gem

If you…or someone you know…is fighting cancer, chances are you're *also* familiar with the debilitating fatigue that often goes hand in hand with the disease. In fact fatigue—the kind that makes it hard to even get out of bed sometimes—is one of the *most* common complaints that cancer sufferers have…and for good reason.

Not only is a cancer patient's body in a *literal* fight for its life, the chemotherapy and radiation treatments that they often must endure can lead to bone-wearying exhaustion. A common side effect of these harsh therapies is a drop in red blood cells (anemia), which causes other cells in the body to not receive enough oxygen and the nutrients they need, like iron or B12, for energy production.

In addition, chemo and radiation produce a number of toxic byproducts that must be detoxified. Not to mention the tremendous amount of harmful molecules known as free radicals that are created which the body must deal with as well.

To make matters even worse weight loss and tissue wasting, known medically as cachexia, is a common problem during cancer treatment and leaves cancer patients feeling spent and weak. And of course we can't overlook the sheer amount of physical and emotional energy that's expended when you're fighting cancer.

Recharge your energy stores naturally

In my practice I combat this fatigue in several different ways. I've had a lot of success with nutritional intravenous therapies. In addition, I've found that supporting the often-overlooked adrenal glands (the stress glands on top of your kidneys) can be tremendously effective. In fact, I think it's *so* important that I'm willing to say that it's an **essential** step in re-energizing those with cancer related fatigue as well as other energy sappers.

This support comes in the form of herbal extracts—known as *adaptogens*—that can help the body and the adrenal glands adapt and cope to physical and mental stress. They have helped thousands of my patients with cancer revitalize over the years. Common ones I use with patients include ashwagandha, rhodiola, and various ginsengs.

But there's one ginseng in particular that's a shining star when it comes to beating cancer fatigue. Researchers have confirmed that one of America's native plants—American ginseng—may be just what's needed for getting over that energy slump.

While many people have heard of the more common Asian ginseng…often referred to as Panax ginseng…few are familiar with the American variety. Also known as Panax quinquefolius, American ginseng is indigenous to the forests of northern and central US. China imports American ginseng where it is highly revered in traditional Chinese medicine. It contains active constituents known as ginsenosides, which support adrenal gland function. These ginsenosides contain nerve relaxing, anti-inflammatory, anti-fatigue, pain relieving, and digestive tonic properties.[1]

American herb helps restore balance

Recently, mainstream researchers confirmed what holistic doctors like myself have already know about herbal adaptogens like American ginseng…and that is that they work! A recent study headed by Mayo clinic, and reported on at the 2012 Annual Meeting of the American Society of Clinical Oncology, found that American ginseng was effective in treating cancer related fatigue.

The study involved 340 patients with cancer who were receiving treatment at one of 40 community medical centers. Sixty percent of the patients had been diagnosed with breast cancer. Participants received

2000 mg of pure American ginseng in capsule form daily or a placebo.

During the first 4 weeks of the study those taking the ginseng had only a slight reduction in their fatigue. However, by week 8 there was a significant improvement in fatigue when they were compared to those taking a placebo. In addition, there were zero side effects found in those taking the ginseng.[2]

When you add these new findings to previous studies using American ginseng that have demonstrated the herb inhibits cancer cell proliferation and tumor growth and this becomes a must-have therapy in my book.[3,4] If you're suffering from cancer related fatigue speak with your holistic doctor or oncologist about using an adaptogen such as American ginseng to help relieve your exhaustion naturally.

Citations:

1. Stengler, Mark. The Natural Physician's Healing Therapies, 2010. Prentice Hall Press. Page 222.

2. 2012 American Society of Clinical Oncology Annual Meeting; "Phase III evaluation of American ginseng (panax quinquefolius) to improve cancer-related fatigue" Debra L. Barton et al. Accessed July 22, 2012 at http://www.asco.org/ASCOv2/Meetings/Abstracts?&vmview=abst_detail_view&confID=114&abstractID=94721

3. Wang CZ, Aung HH, Zhang B, Sun S, Li XL, He H, Xie JT, He TC, Du W, Yuan CS. Chemopreventive effects of heat-processed Panax quinquefolius root on human breast cancer cells. Anticancer Res. 2008 Sep-Oct;28(5A):2545-51.

4. King ML, Murphy LL. American ginseng (Panax quinquefolius L.) extract alters mitogen-activated protein kinase cell signaling and inhibits proliferation of MCF-7 cells. J Exp Ther Oncol. 2007;6(2):147-55

Fish Oil Protects Against Cancer—Not Causes It!

I woke up one morning to a barrage of panicked emails from patients and colleagues asking me to weigh in on a stunning study that seemed to be saying that fish oil could CAUSE prostate cancer. I assured them the study must be bogus and promised to get to the bottom of this clearly outrageous claim. After all, based on a stack of earlier research we already know that the complete opposite is true. In fact, the omega-3 fatty acids in fish and fish-oil supplements *protect* against a variety of cancers and reduce inflammation (a key player in the initiation of cancer). Something smelled fishy here, and I was determined to get to the real truth.

The study that's causing all the uproar is actually an analysis of data from the Selenium and Vitamin E Cancer Prevention Trial, also known as the SELECT trial. Researchers compared the omega-3 blood levels of 834 men who developed prostate cancer over the seven to 12 year span of the trial, to the omega-3 levels in 1,393 men who didn't develop prostate cancer.

The data was then broken down into four groups based on the participants' blood levels of omega-3 and omega-6 fatty acids. The omega-3 blood levels that were examined included plant-derived, short-chain omega-3 fatty acids called ALA. The others were three long-chain omega-3s known as EPA, DPA, and DHA, which are found in seafood. The conclusion of the analysis was that men with the very highest levels of fish oil intake (from food or supplements) had a 71 percent higher risk of high-grade prostate cancer compared with men with the lowest levels.[1]

Females and fish oil

A recent meta-analysis published in the British Medical Journal found that higher levels of omega-3 polyunsaturated fatty acids from seafood are associated with a 14 percent lower risk for breast cancer.[8]

Those are numbers that would grab anyone's attention. But remember when mom used to tell you that you should never judge a book by its cover? She was right. We need to take a close look at what the evidence in this study really tells us.

Digging deeper for the REAL story

First we need to take a look at the previous research on fish oil and prostate cancer. In 2010 McGill University conducted a review of 31 studies and found fish consumption was associated with an impressive 63 percent reduction in the risk for late-stage or fatal prostate cancer.[2] And a study published just this year in the journal of the Canadian Urological Association concluded that the amount of omega-3 and omega-6 fatty acids in your diet "does not significantly affect risk of prostate cancer."[3]

In another study reported in *Cancer Prevention Research*, 48 men who were scheduled to undergo prostate removal due to prostate cancer, were randomly assigned either a low-fat diet with 5 grams of fish oil daily, a diet with an omega-6 to omega-3 ratio of 2:1, or a typical Western diet (control group) where the ratio of omega-6 to omega-3 was 15:1, for four to six weeks before the operation. The researchers found that a low-fat diet with fish oil capsules *slowed* the growth of prostate cancer cells.[4]

So it's clear that there's no lack of evidence refuting the findings of this latest study. But now let's look at what is problematic about the study itself starting with some statistical acrobatics that would make any ringmaster proud.

A study with more holes than Swiss cheese

The authors found a 0.2 percent difference in the proportion of omega-3 fatty acids in red blood cells between the men who developed prostate cancer and those who never developed prostate cancer. Yes, 0.2 percent! And yet, using statistical smokescreens these researchers have managed to unnecessarily frighten men and steering them away from all the PROVEN health benefits of omega-3 fatty acids.

Frankly, I'd expect more from so-called professional scientists. But instead I get more monkey business like this outrageous statement from

Dr. Alan Kristal, the senior author of the paper: "We've shown once again that use of nutritional supplements may be harmful."[5] I wouldn't surprise me one bit if that was a prepared statement written by a Big Pharma PR firm. You know, one of the members of the Drug Club that wants supplements to be available only by prescription so they can charge you sky high drug prices.

Despite countless positive studies proving the benefits of nutritional supplements it seems Dr. Kristal would like us to believe that they are dangerous. Despite the impeccable record nutritional supplements have according to government agencies it would appear that he would rather drum up fear. But the real truth is that this study never assessed whether any of the participants even took fish oil supplements! In fact, the observational review never assessed the source of participants' omega-3 intake at all.

Bad science leads to bad results

But I'm not done with flaws yet, not by a long shot. And the next one is a real doozy. The men's blood was taken just **once** at the **start** of the seven to 12-year study. Needless to say, it's simply just not good science to draw any conclusions about the relationship of prostate cancer and omega fatty acids based on a single seven to 12 year old blood test. It's easy to see how things could go wrong. For example, a man could have had seafood for lunch the day of his blood draw causing a spike in long-chain fatty acid levels. A single test tells us nothing about his average intake of fish-derived omega-3 fatty acids. And to make matters worse, the study used an outdated testing method for measuring blood (plasma) fatty acids levels. The unreliable testing method was developed more than 50 years ago and better technology exists.

Complicating things further, the authors of the study even acknowledged that the men in the study had very low blood concentrations of omega-3s. Common sense tells us that with those low numbers these guys were not likely consumers of fish oil supplements on a regular basis.

Lastly, the data analysis is just plain weird. As Dr. Duffy MacKay from the Council for Responsible Nutrition put it, "If you look at the data… it appears that the non-smokers had more aggressive prostate cancer. It appears that non-drinkers, or people who drank less than one alcoholic drink at baseline, were at a higher risk of prostate cancer… If you listen to this study, you should not only cut omega-3 but you should start smoking cigarettes and drinking more."[6]

Cadillacs and prostate cancer

Dr. Anthony D'Amico, a professor of radiation oncology at Harvard Medical School, and a prostate cancer expert who is known for his work in the detection and treatment of prostate cancer, had some interesting things to say about this study's flaws: "These studies are simply association and when you have an association type study, the way you strengthen it…is that you try to adjust for that association, for all the things you know you can cause prostate cancer. And this is the main issue with the study. They tried this, but they didn't do it properly…they left out some very important risk factors for prostate cancer… The thing that concerns me most is that you can find almost anything associated with aggressive prostate cancer. You can find that driving a Cadillac (could be linked to it)…if you don't adjust for the factors that are known to be associated with it, and you know, from a truly scientific standpoint that's what makes this association extremely weak and possibly false."[7]

Unless some compelling solid research comes out linking fish-derived omega-3s to prostate cancer risk I'm advising my patients to continue eating healthy seafood (for example wild salmon and sardines) and taking a quality fish oil supplement from a maker they trust. As numerous studies have shown, inflammation-fighting fish-derived omega-3s could help protect your brain, heart, skin, and joints. They're good for prenatal health and could help you **win** the battle against cancer.

Article Citations:

1. Brasky TM et al. Plasma Phospholipid Fatty Acids and Prostate Cancer Risk in the SELECT Trial. J Natl Cancer Inst (2013). First published online: July 10, 2013. doi: 10.1093/jnci/djt174. Accessed at http://jnci.oxfordjournals.org/content/early/2013/07/09/jnci.djt174

2. Szymanski KM, et al. Fish consumption and prostate cancer risk: a review and meta-analysis. Am J Clin Nutr. 2010 Nov;92(5):1223-33. doi: 10.3945/ajcn.2010.29530. Epub 2010 Sep 15. Review.

3. Chua ME, et al. The relevance of serum levels of long chain omega-3 polyunsaturated fatty acids and prostate cancer risk: A meta-analysis. Can Urol Assoc J. 2013 May;7(5-6):E333-43. doi: 10.5489/cuaj.1056.

4. Aronson WJ, et al. Phase II prospective randomized trial of a low-fat diet with fish oil supplementation in men undergoing radical prostatectomy. Cancer Prev Res (Phila). 2011 Dec;4(12):2062-71. doi: 10.1158/1940-6207.CAPR-11-0298. Epub 2011 Oct 25.

5. KomoNews.com. Accessed July 14, 2013 at http://www.komonews.com/news/health/Fatty-fish-fish-oil-linked-to-increased-prostate-cancer-risk-215094431.html

6. Nutraingredients website. Accessed July 14, 2013 at http://www.nutraingredients.com/Research/Experts-slam-omega-3-link-to-prostate-cancer-as-overblown-scaremongering

7. Ruth, Alan. Nutraingredients.com website. Accessed July 17, 2013 at http://www.nutraingredients.com/On-your-radar/Omega-3/Not-just-industry-slamming-omega-3-prostate-cancer-links?nocount

8. Ju-Sheng Zheng, PhD, et al. Intake of fish and marine n-3 polyunsaturated fatty acids and risk of breast cancer: meta-analysis of data from 21 independent prospective cohort studies. BMJ 2013;346:f3706

Chamomile Tea Benefits Turn Off Cancer Cells

Chamomile compound fights cancer

There's nothing quite like a piping hot cup of tea at the end of a long and hectic day — and if that tea happens to be chamomile, you're not just getting a warm mug of liquid relaxation.

You're getting a ton of chamomile tea benefits and a powerful ally in the fight against cancer.

Cancer cells have what's considered a superpower, at least on a cellular level: They just don't die the way other cells do. They live much longer, allowing tumors to grow, and cancers to spread.

Well, it's time for that superpower to meet its kryptonite — a natural substance called apigenin that's found in abundance in chamomile. In a series of experiments on breast cancer cells, apigenin was able to correct the defect that gives cancer cells their super longevity.

Once corrected, the cells died like normal cells, according to the study of apigenin and chamomile tea benefits in the *Proceedings of the National Academy of Sciences.*

Out in the real world, cancer cells that live and die like normal cells are easy to defeat. And in some cases, they might not have the chance to form a tumor at all — which is why this discovery could pave the way for a natural treatment that could work alongside current therapies or even fight the disease on its own.

And since up to 80 percent of all cancers survive and grow thanks to this same "superpower," the benefits almost certainly won't be limited to the breast cancer cells used in the new study.

I'll keep you posted on this as the research continues to unfold. But in the meantime, you may be able to get the bulk of the chamomile tea benefits right now just by drinking a cup or two each day.

As I wrote in my book _The Natural Physician's Healing Therapies_, there are two forms of chamomile used medicinally, German and Roman. I prefer German because it's less likely to be contaminated with pesticides and other chemicals.

I find it works best when you brew it fresh, but it's also available in other forms — including capsules, tinctures, skin creams, and more. And along with protecting you from cancer, chamomile tea benefits can also fight infection, stress, ulcers, and stomach problems such as irritable bowels, cramps, and flatulence.

But if you're just looking for a source of cancer-fighting apigenin and chamomile isn't your cup of tea, you can also find it in celery and parsley.

CHAPTER 3

The **Secret** Sinister Cause of Heart Disease and Cancer **REVEALED**

For years conventional and holistic doctors have been measuring a blood marker known as C-reactive protein or CRP. The reason is that this protein, produced by the liver, *reflects* the amount of inflammation occurring in the body. And we know that chronic inflammation is associated with almost every chronic disease from cancer to arthritis, diabetes to heart disease, macular degeneration to osteoporosis, and more. When your body is in a state of chronic inflammation it leads to immune system dysfunction and cell/organ destruction. So the level of CRP on a blood test lets you know what your general level of inflammation is. An ideal value is less than 1.0 mg/L.

Going where no test has gone before

Like many things in medicine, laboratory testing is constantly progressing. And while CRP has been helpful in identifying acute and chronic inflammation, there's another blood marker that helps us peer into the world of inflammation. And it's one your doctor might not have even heard of before. The marker has a kind of futuristic Star Trek sounding name. It's known as galectin-3. Galectins include a group of proteins that bind to carbohydrates (molecules containing long sugar chains) known as beta-galactosides. Galectins play an important role both inside and outside of human cells.

So far there have been 15 different types of galectins identified. And we now know that galectin-3 plays an important role in inflammation and our body's immune response. More specifically it *promotes* inflammation, fibrosis (excess fibrous connective tissue in an organ or tissue), kidney disease, obesity, and cancer metastasis. And as it turns out, it's an excellent marker for cardiovascular risk such as heart failure.

Remember I said earlier that CRP *reflects* inflammation in the body? Well galectin-3 is somewhat different. Instead of just *reflecting* inflammation galectin-3 is actually a direct marker of it. And since it's involved in creating the inflammatory response it can be a better *predictor* of the outcome of a disease. This is so important because it means that doctors like me that practice preventative medicine can use the marker to see how well our interventions are working and to adjust our approach. In other words, we can try to head diseases like cancer and heart disease off at the pass and keep them from getting worse.

Helping to head off heart problems

Now let's look at some of the research behind galectin-3 and heart health. One study that caught the attention of the medical world, well some cardiologists at least, was the 2011 PREVEND study. This study— made up of over 8,000 people—spanned approximately 10 years. And it looked at the association between galectin-3 levels in the blood and risk factors for cardiovascular disease.

The researchers found that higher galectin-3 levels were associated with increased mortality rates.[1] And ongoing research confirmed that that an elevated level of galectin-3 is a good predictor of heart failure.[2]

If you have heart disease, galectin-3 is an FDA cleared blood test and your cardiologist may use it to monitor the progression of your disease. Knowing your blood levels of galectin-3 can help with the following:

Frequency of doctor visits—Knowing your galectin-3 levels will help your cardiologist determine the frequency of your follow up visits. If you have an elevated galectin-3 level you will likely need more frequent visits to be monitored properly.

Hospital discharge—If you have an elevated galectin-3 level you are more likely to be re-admitted to the hospital. And if you are *already* in the hospital a high level can help your doctor determine when you are ready for discharge.

Referrals—Your general practitioner, family doctor, or other specialist can use galectin-3 to determine if you are at risk for heart failure related problems and make timely referrals to a cardiologist if you are.

Evaluate treatment options—Your galectin-3 level can help your doctor determine if you need advanced heart failure treatments such as implanted heart defibrillators, pacemakers, or surgery. And it will help your holistic doctor determine what natural therapies will work best. (See the sidebar for more on this.)

The cancer connection

But the benefits of knowing and understanding your galectin-3 levels don't stop at heart health...not by a long shot. In fact, studies have shown that galectin-3 has a diverse involvement in the *formation* of cancer. For example, it is involved in the clumping and migration of cancer cells to tissue, the formation of blood vessels that feed tumors, the prevention of cancer cell death, and the metastasis (spreading) of cancer.[3] And it also helps cancer cells survive chemotherapy treatment. In other words, elevated galectin-3 is bad news if you have cancer.

Of course pharmaceutical companies are doing research on patentable ways to block the effects of galectin-3 for cancer prevention and treatment. But the good news is that we *already* have a natural, non-toxic substance that accomplishes this. It is a nutritional supplement known as modified citrus pectin (MCP).

Know your natural options

Your holistic doctor has a number of natural options available for treating your heart disease and knowing your galectin-3 levels will help him make the choice that's best for you. This includes therapies such as enhanced external counterpulsation (EECP). EECP uses mechanical cuffs that gently but firmly compress the blood vessels in the lower limbs to increase blood flow to your heart allowing your heart to pump blood more easily and efficiently. Your doctor may also use heart specific nutritional supplements such as coenzyme Q10, L carnitine, magnesium, hawthorn extract, ribose, and taurine.

Conquering cancer with citrus

MCP is derived from pectin, which is extracted from the peel and pith (the white threadlike part between a citrus fruit and its peel) of citrus fruits—and is also found in the peel and core of other fruits, such as apples. But the problem with pectin is that in its straight-from-the-fruit state its molecules are just too large for us to digest.

So even if we were to suddenly start chowing down on citrus peels we wouldn't be able to benefit from the pectin. But researcher Isaac Eliaz MD solved this "big molecule" problem by developing a smaller form that can be absorbed and concentrated in a supplement.

MCP actively helps to fight cancer in a number of powerful ways including:

- Binding and interfering with the activity of galectin-3 fighting cancer on several fronts including: preventing tumors from metastasizing.[4]

- Blocking galectin-3's ability to stimulate the formation of blood vessels in new tumors (known as anti-angiogenesis).[5]

- Inducing cancer cell death (*apoptosis*) by interfering with important signaling pathways related to cancer cell proliferation and survival.[6]

- Aiding chemotherapy helping it do its job more effectively.[7]

- Improving immune cell activity.

- Helping reduce heavy metals in the body including lead and mercury, both of which are considered cancer causing agents.[8,9]

Time to get tested

If you have heart disease or cancer you should speak with your doctors about testing your galectin-3. Knowing your blood levels will allow your medical team to access your level of inflammation or cancer progression.

If you have cancer, especially breast or prostate cancer, work with your oncologist and holistic practitioners to incorporate modified citrus pectin into your program. A typical dosage is 5 grams two to three times daily with meals. The brand I recommend is PectaSol-C, a proprietary formulation developed and manufactured by EcoNugenics.

Citations:

1. de Boer RA, van Veldhuisen DJ, Gansevoort RT, Muller Kobold AC, van Gilst WH, Hillege HL, Bakker SJ, van der Harst P. The fibrosis marker galectin-3 and outcome in the general population. J Intern Med. 2012 Jul;272(1):55-64. doi: 10.1111/j.1365-2796.2011.02476.x. Epub 2011 Nov 18.

2. Grandin EW, Jarolim P, Murphy SA, Ritterova L, Cannon CP, Braunwald E, Morrow DA. Galectin-3 and the development of heart failure after acute coronary syndrome: pilot experience from PROVE IT-TIMI 22. Clin Chem. 2012 Jan;58(1):267-73. Epub 2011 Nov 22.

3. Nangia-Makker P, Balan V, Raz A. Galectin-3 binding and metastasis.Methods Mol Biol. 2012;878:251-66.

4. Glinsky VV, Raz A.Modified citrus pectin anti-metastatic properties: one bullet, multiple targets. Carbohydr Res. 2009 Sep 28;344(14):1788-91. Epub 2008 Sep 26.

5. Nangia-Makker P, Hogan V, Honjo Y, Baccarini S, Tait L, Bresalier R, Raz A. Inhibition of human cancer cell growth and metastasis in nude mice by oral intake of modifiedcitrus pectin. J Natl Cancer Inst. 2002 Dec 18;94(24):1854-62.

6. Tehranian N, Sepehri H, Mehdipour P, Biramijamal F, Hossein Nozhad A, Sarrafnejad A, Hajizadeh E. Combination effect of PectaSol and Doxorubicin on viability, cell cycle arrest and apoptosis in DU-145 and LNCaP prostate cancer cell lines. Cell Biol Int. 2012 Jul;36(7):601-10.

7. Ramachandran C, Wilk BJ, Hotchkiss A, Chau H, Eliaz I, Melnick SJ. Activation of human T-helper/inducer cell, T-cytotoxic cell, B-cell, and natural killer (NK)-cells and induction of natural killer cell activity against K562 chronic myeloid leukemia cells with modified citrus pectin. BMC Complement Altern Med. 2011 Aug 4;11:59.

8. Zhao ZY, Liang L, Fan X, Yu Z, Hotchkiss AT, Wilk BJ. The Role of Modified Citrus Pectin as an Effective Chelator of Lead in Children Hospitalized with Toxic Lead Levels. Altern Ther Health Med.2008 14(4):34-8

9. Eliaz I, Hotchkiss AT, Fishman ML, Rode D. The Effect of Modified Citrus Pectin on Urinary Excretion of Toxic Elements. Phytother Res.2006 20(10):859-64.

CHAPTER 4

Stay Away from These **Cancer-Causing** Prescription Drugs

How your statin drug may make you 15 times more likely to get cancer

Last month I warned you about the big diabetes risk that statin users face. Amazingly, most of my patients–not to mention most doctors I know—knew nothing about this huge risk until I told them. Even though the research has been published in major medical journals. Talk about mainstream suppression!

But it gets even worse. It doesn't stop at raising the risk of getting diabetes by up to 80 percent. No, instead, new research links statin drugs to an increased cancer risk. (Maybe that revelation will *finally* get doctors to stop shoving it down patients' throats.)

Oh, and in case you were wondering the answer is "no." This data does not come from some unknown trade publication or anti-medicine website. In fact it was reported at a recent American College of Cardiology conference. And honestly, that's just about as mainstream as you can get.

Cholesterol plays an important roles in human health, and despite what we've been told by the pharmaceutical companies, achieving the lowest possible amount of serum cholesterol is not desirable or beneficial. In fact, researchers from Tufts found that modestly lower LDL levels may point to a higher risk for cancer.

The group from Tufts Medical Center in Boston looked at data from the Framingham Heart Study of 5,124 adults not taking statins. Doctors followed up with the volunteers every four years for 18 years. They found that having lower serum LDL was linked with higher cancer risk.[1]

And this research is not the first to link statins and cancer. Incredibly, an earlier study found low LDL levels (equal to or below 70 mg/dL) make you 15 times more likely to get a blood cancer![2]

Research proves statins don't make you live longer

Sure…statin drugs lower your liver's production of cholesterol and can lower your cholesterol numbers. But do they really extend your life? No, not according to a meta-analysis of 65,000 people published in *Evidence Based Medicine*. Researchers found no link between using a statin drug and living longer. As a matter of fact, it didn't find any relationship between cholesterol levels and survival rates. Even more disturbing, a number of studies have linked lower cholesterol levels to *higher* death rates.[3] So taking a statin could actually be putting you at greater risk of dying.

Your body needs LDL cholesterol—or you wouldn't have it

Most doctors insist that the lower your LDL cholesterol, the better. But the research proves that it doesn't keep you alive any longer and it could cause other serious health problems as well.

And the reason why is quite simple.

You see our Creator gave us LDL cholesterol as part of many important roles in the body. We NEED it to be healthy. LDL cholesterol fuels and protects our cells by moving essential fatty acids and fat-soluble vitamins, including A, D, E, K, and the vitamin-like CoQ10, around the body. These antioxidants are needed for brain function, energy production, to protect our cells from damage, balance our blood sugar, control inflammation, and bone growth, and to support our immune system.

Benefits of apples better than statins
Nature's answer to cholesterol meds

Forget statins. If you want to protect your ticker, prevent a heart attack, stop a stroke, stay healthy and enjoy a great snack all at the same time, bite into a crisp, juicy apple.

Yes... an apple. Call it nature's original wonder drug.

One new study out of the prestigious Oxford University compares the benefits of statins to the benefits of apples. Do I even need to tell you which one comes out on top?

Apples, of course.

Since the researchers were British, they used UK numbers. They estimated that if everyone in the nation over the age of 50 was offered statins — as some would just love to see happen — and 70 percent of them actually took the drugs, the number of vascular deaths would drop by 9,400 per year.

A life saved is a life saved, I won't argue otherwise.

But in this case, those lives saved would come at a terrible cost: The drugs would also cause 10,000 new cases of diabetes and 1,000 new cases of muscle disease (and leave countless others suffering from other statin side effects, including memory loss, kidney and liver problems and sexual dysfunction).

Giving those same over-50s apples instead of drugs, on the other hand, would save almost as many lives and come with none of the risks. In fact, helping to prevent diabetes, not cause it, is one of the added benefits of apples– and that's not the only science at the core of this issue.

One study I told you about recently shows apples truly are nature's answer to statins, cutting LDL cholesterol levels by as much as 40 percent in just one month.

Apples can also raise HDL ("good") cholesterol, and eating them regularly can help you to feel full so you're less likely to overeat — potentially helping you to lose weight.

The only downside is that conventional apples have topped the Environmental Working Group's "dirty dozen" list for three years running — and that's not an honor.

That's a list of fruit and vegetables most likely to be contaminated with pesticides. And with apples, studies have shown that the chemicals can penetrate the skin and enter the fruit — so you can get dosed even if you wash and peel it.

Go organic instead to get all of the benefits of apples without any added pesticides. You'll pay a little more, but it'll be worth every penny.

And they can't do any of it without LDL.

LDL cholesterol also fights infections like *Staphylococcus aureus*, the bacteria responsible for the frightening flesh-eating disease that was all over the news a few years ago. In fact, the same study I mentioned above that showed the jump in blood cancer risk *also* found those with low LDL cholesterol had a big increase in their risk for severe infections.[4]

Studies, like the one published in the *Journal of Gerontology* last year, also show that LDL cholesterol is needed to build and maintain muscles.[5] And if you're older this is critical because as we age we lose muscle mass.

And what the mainstream always ignores is that LDL levels can warn us if something *is* wrong. Just like a fever warns us when we have an infection having LDL levels that are too high or too low can tell us something is out of balance in our body. When we find and correct that underlying problem your LDL levels should return to normal.

It's time to get rid of the idea that LDL is "bad" or the enemy. With cholesterol, like most things in life, it's all about balance.

Article Citations:

1. American College of Cardiology 2012; Abstract 911-7. "The association between lower levels of low-density lipoprotein cholesterol and cancer predates the diagnosis of cancer by 18 years"

2. Annals of Clinical and Laboratory Science, 2007; 37(4):343-8. "Low serum LDL cholesterol levels and the risk of fever, sepsis, and malignancy."

3. Evidence Based Medicine. 2011;16(1):8-9. "Statins are not associated with a decrease in all cause mortality in a high-risk primary prevention setting."

4. Annals of Clinical and Laboratory Science, 2007; 37(4):343-8. "Low serum LDL cholesterol levels and the risk of fever, sepsis, and malignancy."

5. "'Bad' cholesterol not as bad as people think, study shows." Texas A&M University (2011, May 5). ScienceDaily

The Shocking Truth About How Your Blood Pressure Medication Could Give You Cancer!

Imagine finding out that a medication that you've been taking for years can more than double the risk of developing cancer!

Unfortunately, for many women who are on one popular drug, they don't have to imagine, the nightmare is very real. This was the shocking conclusion of a new study published in the *Journal of the American Medical Association Internal Medicine*.[1]

The new research confirms that a common class of blood pressure medications called calcium channel blockers can send your breast cancer risk skyrocketing by two and half times or more. And when I say common I really mean it… they account for approximately 100 million prescriptions a year.

The list of drugs in this group includes amlodipine (Norvasc), diltiazem (Cardizem LA, Tiazac), isradipine (DynaCirc CR), nicardipine (Cardene SR), nifedipine (Procardia, Procardia XL, Adalat CC), nisoldipine (Sular), and verapamil (Calan, Verelan, Covera-PM).

Older women, who have been on the drugs for more than 10 years had the highest risk. And when you consider that channel blockers are one of those "set it and forget drugs" that doctors tend to leave their patients on for a lifetime, that means that a staggering number of women are at risk.

After ten years the women in the study on calcium channel blockers saw their lobular cancer risk leap up to 2.6 times that of the volunteers who had never taken the drugs. And their risk of ductal breast cancer wasn't far behind, skyrocketing to 2.4 times that of the non-drug-takers.

Other blood pressure medications showed no association with breast cancer. But they, of course, come with plenty of potential side effects of their own.

More research is needed, but these findings are already very alarming. I suggest working with a holistic doctor to transition over to natural hypertension treatments and work towards getting rid of the drugs altogether.

Article Citation:
1. Patricia F. Coogan, Patricia F Calcium-Channel Blockers and Breast CancerA Hypothesis Revived. JAMA Internal Medicine.August 5, 2013.

CHAPTER 5

How to Prevent Prostate Cancer

Common prostate drugs given to millions linked to aggressive prostate cancer

There are lots of good things about getting older. With age comes wisdom, which means as we pack more birthdays under our belt we're much more confident in ourselves and our decisions. Plus studies show that contrary to the grumpy old person stereotype, as we get older we're actually much more content and satisfied with our lives. And with kids grown-up and moving out of the house you might suddenly find yourself with the extra time you always wanted to pursue hobbies and just relax.

But if you're a guy there's one thing that often comes with age that's anything but welcome. I'm talking about prostate problems. In fact, having an enlarged prostate…a condition known as benign prostatic hyperplasia (BPH)…is so common that there are currently millions of men taking prescription drugs to treat the problem. Doctors prescribe

The PSA coin toss

PSA is not a great test for prostate cancer screening. In fact, in 2010 Richard Ablin, PhD, the researcher who discovered PSA in 1970, has stated that the PSA test is a "hugely expensive public health disaster" and "hardly more effective than a coin toss."[3] Indeed two large studies recently published in the New England Journal of Medicine demonstrated that "PSA screening had either no or little effect on the death rate from prostate cancer."[4] To be fair there is some usefulness for the PSA test. Ablin confirms that the PSA test can be useful in monitoring men who had treatment for prostate cancer.[5] Also, consistent increases in PSA levels (known as PSA velocity) may indicate prostate cancer, although the research in this area is inconclusive.

these drugs to shrink the prostate and help improve bothersome symptoms including night-time urination, weak stream, urgency to urinate, leaking, and incomplete bladder emptying.

The shocking link between prostate drugs and prostate cancer

Unfortunately, it turns out that those millions of men may be unknowingly trading their bothersome prostate symptoms for something much, much worse. Shockingly, research has now revealed that BPH drugs increase your risk of developing an *aggressive* form of prostate cancer! Most men develop some form of prostate cancer if they live long enough. Fortunately most are slow growing and do not kill. The concern is that the aggressive forms can spread quickly to vital organs of the body and become fatal.

In two large trials the link between 5-alpha reductase inhibitors (5-ARIs) and this form of prostate cancer was so strong that, in a rare move, the FDA actually mandated a change to the drug labels. Specifically, the labels must now carry a warning about the increased risk of being diagnosed with a more serious form of prostate cancer.[1] These medications include Proscar (finasteride), Avodart (dutasteride), and Jalyn (dutasteride and tamsulosin). This warning also extends to the popular medication Propecia used for male pattern hair loss, because it contains a low dose of finasteride.

5-ARIs inhibit the enzyme that converts the male hormone into dihydrotestosterone (DHT). DHT is one of the hormones thought to stimulate prostate enlargement. And the drugs have been shown to reduce the overall risk of prostate cancer. Sounds good so far, right? But the paradox of these medications is that at the same time they *increase* the risk of more serious, aggressive prostate cancers. No doubt this is a scary trade-off.

As a reader of *Health Revelations* you're probably already aware that PSA is not a great test for identifying prostate cancer. (See pages 46-47 for more on this.) But, unfortunately many doctors still mistakenly rely on this number alone as an indicator. In these cases a diagnosis may be delayed because 5-alpha reductase inhibitors could be masking the cancer since they can reduce prostate specific antigen (PSA) blood values by approximately 50 percent.[2] So, in other words, a man taking these drugs could have a normal PSA level *despite* having an aggressive prostate cancer forming.

If you're taking one of these drugs and want to continue with them I recommend that you request prostate ultrasound testing in addition to blood work and a yearly digital prostate exam. This combination of approaches can help your doctor catch any potentially aggressive forms of cancer earlier. The better long-term choice, of course, is working with a doctor skilled in natural medicine who can help you take advantage of nature's nontoxic remedies to relieve your troubling BPH symptoms. My patients find they work well.

Reduce PSA levels and heal your prostate naturally

Recent research published in the *British Journal of Nutrition* found that omega-3 fatty acids and coenzyme Q10 significantly lowered PSA levels in healthy men. The study involved 504 men who were randomly assigned to receive 400 mg of coenzyme Q10, omega-3 (4.48 grams of EPA and 2.88 grams of DHA), 2400 mg of gamma-linolenic acid (GLA), or a placebo daily for 12 weeks. Those taking the omega-3 and coenzyme Q10 supplements had a 30 percent and 33 percent reduction in their PSA levels, respectively. Those taking GLA had an increased level of PSA by about 15 percent.[6]

I regularly recommend omega-3 supplements and omega-3 rich foods to my male patients because they reduce prostate inflammation and swelling. Diets that are rich in omega-3s, such as the Mediterranean diet, have a protective effect against a variety of different cancers, including cancer of the prostate. And of course omega-3 fatty acids benefit many other parts of the body—including the brain, joints, skin, heart and arteries, and immune system to name just a few. Good food sources of omega-3 are flaxseed and fish including salmon, sardines, and trout.

In the same *BJN* study GLA was shown to *increase* PSA levels. GLA is a type of fatty acid that comes from the omega-6 family of fatty

Miracle Mineral Could Reduce Your Risk of Prostate Cancer by Forty Percent or More!

Utter the words prostate cancer and most men are filled with dread. And for good reason, after all we've all heard the horror stories… impotence, incontinence, or worse. But I can usually get a guy to crack a smile when I explain that a very inexpensive mineral could significantly reduce his risk of ever getting aggressive prostate cancer in the first place.

Now holistic doctors like me have known for quite some time that people with higher levels of selenium in their blood have lower rates of death from cancer, including the prostate variety. But what has remained unclear however, is just how much selenium you need on board to avoid getting prostate cancer. With the goal of figuring out that level, researchers in the United Kingdom looked at a number of studies (a meta-analysis) that included reported measurements of selenium intake or status (plasma, serum, or toenail selenium), assessments of prostate cancer cases (number of events), and the relative risk (the risk of developing the disease relative to exposure) in the adult population.

Prostate cancer risk plummeted

Using sophisticated statistical analyses, the researchers determined that blood concentrations of selenium between 135 and 170 ng/mL reduced the risk of an aggressive form of prostate cancer by up to 40 percent![1] Your doctor can order your blood selenium level with any of the standard laboratories.

Selenium is a "trace mineral." But don't make the mistake of thinking that it's of limited importance. The truth is the human body requires small, or trace, amounts of the mineral to function. Selenium is actually essential for life. It's required for the proper functioning of a number of enzyme systems in the body which control cell metabolism. Some examples include the proper functioning of glutathione—your body's master antioxidant—as well as other antioxidant systems in the body. Selenium is also needed to produce the most powerful thyroid hormone in the body known as triiodothyronine (T3). And it's a key nutrient involved in ridding your body of toxins including carcinogens.

Low selenium levels linked to weakened immunities

Selenium deficiency contributes to a weakened immune system. According to the Linus Pauling Institute at Oregon State University, "There is a great deal of evidence indicating that selenium supplementation at high levels reduces the incidence of cancer in animals. More than two-thirds of over 100 published studies in 20 different animal models of spontaneous, viral, and chemically induced cancers found that selenium supplementation significantly reduces tumor incidence."[2]

Other studies have shown a link between low dietary selenium intake and prostate cancer risk. For example, a large prospective study published in the Journal of the National Cancer Institute involved over 30,000 male health professionals in the United States. Toenail selenium samples were tested and researchers found higher selenium levels were associated with a significantly reduced risk of advanced prostate cancer.[3]

It's best to raise your selenium through diet

They also found that men with toenail selenium content consistent with an average daily dietary intake of 159 mcg/day of selenium had a 65% lower risk of advanced prostate cancer compared to those with toenail selenium content consistent with an average intake of 86 mcg/day.[4]

As with most nutrients, it's best to raise your selenium through diet. Good food sources of selenium include:

- Brazil nuts—3 nuts contains approximately 270 micrograms

- Sardines—3 ounces contains approximately 50 mcg

- Halibut—4 ounces contains approximately 50 mcg

- Eggs—1 egg contains approximately 15 mcg

- Brown rice—1 cup contains approximately 19 mcg

- Sunflower seeds—quarter cup contains approximately 19 mcg

A good daily intake of selenium for adults is 200 micrograms. You can get this through diet and supplementation if needed. The upper limit for selenium intake is 400 micrograms daily. Remember that more is not better when it comes to trace minerals like selenium. Excessive selenium intake can cause side effects; although research shows this requires significantly higher levels than 400 micrograms. Talk with your doctor about measuring your own levels and determining how much you need.

Prostate cancer affects 1 in 6 men in the United States. A diet that consistently includes selenium rich foods is one of the best ways for men to stave off this all too common disease.

Article Citations:

1. Hurst R, et al. Selenium and prostate cancer: systematic review and meta-analysis. Am J Clin Nutr 2012;96(1): 111 122.

2. Combs GF, Jr., Gray WP. Chemopreventive agents: selenium. Pharmacol Ther. 1998;79(3):179-192.

3. Yoshizawa K, Willett WC, Morris SJ, et al. Study of prediagnostic selenium level in toenails and the risk of advanced prostate cancer. J Natl Cancer Inst. 1998;90(16):1219-1224.

4. ibid

acids. When you get too many omega-6 fats in your diet it encourages inflammation and it's believed to increase your risk for a variety of inflammatory health conditions including cancer. Another study, published in the journal *Nutrition Research*, concluded that "a high dietary ratio of (omega-6 to omega-3) fatty acids may increase the risk of overall prostate cancer among white men and possibly increase the risk of high-grade prostate cancer among all men."[7] Americans typically get way too many omega-6 fatty acids in their diet in the form of vegetable oils, processed packaged food, and restaurant meals. Reducing the omega-6s in your diet could help reduce your cancer risks.

Make your diet prostate-friendly

Prostate health is greatly influenced by what you put in your mouth. Red meat, dairy products, and animal fat are all associated with prostate cancer.[8] I believe refined sugar products—which includes most bread—should be added to that list as well.

The prostate is very sensitive to hormones. These foods can increase the levels of male hormones and growth hormones in the body leading to prostate enlargement and even cancer. So for a healthy prostate it's best to cut back on *all* of them. And when you do choose to eat them make sure you're picking hormone-free organic products.

Better yet, just slash animal-derived proteins from your diet entirely if you can manage it…except for organic eggs and cold water fish such as salmon, sardines, or trout. Instead focus on protein-rich plant sources such as beans, lentils, pumpkin seeds, and quinoa. This will help reduce inflammation and growth of the prostate.

The truth about soy and prostates

I'm often asked what I think about soy foods and their effect on the prostate. Many clinicians tell patients that soy is "bad" for the prostate because it contains phytoestrogens—naturally occurring chemicals in plants that mimic the hormone estrogen. The reality is that there are a stack of studies showing just the opposite. Soy consumption by men is associated with a *reduction* in prostate cancer![9]

It turns out that phytoestrogens can inhibit the growth of various cancers. One well-studied compound found in soy is genistein. Genistein has been shown to reduce prostate cancer cell activity. According to the National Cancer Institute, " Several laboratory studies have found that treating human prostate cancer cells with isoflavones (such as genistein or daidzein) interferes with pathways in prostate cancer cells related to inflammation and cancer growth and spread."[10]

Unfortunately, most of the soy available in the U.S. has been highly processed with solvents to the remove soy oil from the bean. And even worse, most of it has been genetically modified so the chemicals they provide are different from what our bodies were designed for. In the Far East soy is consumed as a whole food no matter whether it's cooked, roasted, fermented, or sprouted. Eating just two ounces of fermented soy foods a couple of times a week can have a protective effect. Fermented soy products include tempeh, tofu, natto, and soy miso.

Prostate-cancer fighters from the produce aisle

Men who eat lots of vegetables have a lower risk of prostate enlargement and prostate cancer. But fitting in the five to seven servings of vegetables a day you need to protect yourself against cancer can be quite a challenge. An easy way to sneak more veggies into your diet… and a trick I use myself…is to drop an assortment of vegetables into the blender each morning with a protein drink mix and some unsweetened coconut or almond milk. I like to include carrots, beets, zucchini, and romaine lettuce along with several cancer-crushing cruciferous veggies like broccoli, cauliflower, Brussels sprouts, cabbage, bok choy, collard greens, and kale.

Vegetables are naturally rich in immune-enhancing nutrients, including carotenoids and vitamins C, E, and K. They also contain compounds known as glucosinolates, which are converted into the anti-cancer compounds indole 3, carbinol, and sulforaphane in the body. These nutrients help the liver break down estrogen, a hormone that stimulates prostate growth when levels are too high (which is often the case in overweight men).

Prostate healer from the Middle East

Pomegranate trees are a common sight in the Middle East, Israel, and Iran. But it wasn't until the late 1700's that the fruit tree made it to North America. Today the pomegranate has become quite popular and you can get it in most grocery stores. But the benefits of the fruit go well beyond its snacking potential. It turns out that the delicious pomegranate may also be a cancer fighter.

Test tube studies show that pomegranate causes cancer cell death and inhibits blood flow to tumors.[11,12] An interesting study out of UCLA looked at the effect of pomegranate in men who had radiation or surgery for prostate cancer. Researchers found that when these men were given 8 ounces of pomegranate juice daily the time it took their PSA levels to double (a common measurement that doctors use to judge how a prostate problem is progressing) became *significantly* longer. In addition, there was a drop in the growth of cancer cells and a spike in cancer cells dying off.[13]

As a side benefit, pomegranate juice has been shown to improve erectile dysfunction by improving penile blood flow.[14] Aim to drink two to eight ounces of the juice a day or to eat a fresh pomegranate several times a week to promote prostate health.

Protect your prostate with ketchup

Hidden inside tomatoes and some other pink and red fruits is a powerful prostate-friendly nutrient called lycopene. Lycopene is a type of carotenoid or pigment that provides tomatoes with their deep red color. It's also found in watermelon, pink grapefruit, and guava.

German researchers found elderly men with benign prostatic hyperplasia who were given 15 mg lycopene supplements had their PSA levels drop. Along with that drop the men's prostates stopped growing. The PSA levels of the men who were given a placebo, however, didn't budge and their prostates continued to grow.[15]

Several studies have linked lycopene-rich foods to a reduction in prostate cancer risk. In fact, just one serving a day has been shown to have a protective effect. Your body is able to use more lycopene from the foods you eat if the cell walls of the food are broken down. So choose foods like tomato juice, ketchup, and tomato sauces (organic, of course) to make sure you're getting the most benefit.

Kill cancer cells and suppress inflammation with common spices

You may already have a bottle of this cancer-fighter in your kitchen cabinet. I'm talking about the delicious golden yellow spice turmeric. Several studies show that eating turmeric lowers the risk of a variety of cancers, including prostate. Turmeric has a unique ability to suppress inflammation and keep cancer cells from multiplying. Make it a goal to use a teaspoonful with meals a couple times a week. It's also available as a supplement.

Turmeric isn't the only spice-rack staple that could play a role in keeping your prostate healthy. If you're a fan of spicy foods you're sure to be familiar with fiery cayenne. You may even be familiar with the spice's medicinal use a topical pain reliever and as a circulation-booster when eaten. But you probably never realized that it may also play an important role in prostate health.

Research has shown that cayenne induces prostate cancer cell death.[16] Researchers from Nottingham University found it destroys the mitochondria (energy producing factory) of cancer cells.[17] You can add a pinch of cayenne to your dishes to spice up meal time and protect your prostate at the same time. And if your taste buds lean towards the mild side you can pick up the spice as a supplement instead. Cayenne has a blood-thinning effect so be sure to check with your doctor before using large amounts of the spice.

Top it all off with the right tea

Tea is a known cancer fighter. But too much caffeine can be irritating to the prostate and bladder, which means for some men tea can make urinating more difficult. Your best bet is to pick a green tea, which will have significantly less caffeine but is still loaded with the anti-cancer and anti-inflammatory compounds you want.

There are many studies that show that regularly drinking green tea—generally three to five cups or more a day—has a protective effect against prostate cancer. Green tea is rich in powerful antioxidants known as polyphenols. The most important is EGCG. These antioxidants protect against damage to cell DNA (genetic material that controls cell replication), cause cancer cells to stop replicating, improve immunity, and support the liver's ability to rid the body of cancer-causing compounds. I recommend picking an *organic* green tea, which is readily available in most supermarkets and health food stores.

Sources:

1. FDA website. Accessed January 1, 2013 at www.fda.gov/Drugs/DrugSafety/ucm258314.htm

2. ibid

3. Medscape Today website. Accessed January 1, 2013 at www.medscape.com/viewarticle/718351

4. ibid

5. ibid

6. Safarinejad M. R. et al. Effects of EPA, gamma-linolenic acid or coenzyme Q10 on serum prostate-specific antigen levels: a randomised, double-blind trial. British Journal of Nutrition. Published online December 2012.

7. Williams CD, Whitley BM, Hoyo C, Grant DJ, Iraggi JD, Newman KA, Gerber L, Taylor LA, McKeever MG, Freedland SJ., A high ratio of dietary n-6/n-3 polyunsaturated fatty acids is associated with increased risk of prostate cancer. Nutr Res. 2011 Jan;31(1):1-8. doi: 10.1016/j.nutres.2011.01.002.

8. Key TJ, Schatzkin A, Willett WC, Allen NE, Spencer EA, Travis RC. Diet, nutrition and the prevention of cancer. Public Health Nutr. 2004 Feb;7(1A):193.

9. Yan L, Spitznagel EL. Soy consumption and prostate cancer risk in men: a revisit of a meta-analysis. Am J Clin Nutr. 2009 Apr;89(4):1155-63. doi: 10.3945/ajcn.2008.27029. Epub 2009 Feb 11.

10. National Cancer Institute website. Accessed January 5, 2013 at www.cancer.gov/cancertopics/pdq/cam/prostatesupplements/Patient/page7

11. Seeram NP et al. In vitro antiproliferative, apoptotic and antioxidant activities of punicalagin, ellagic acid and a total pomegranate tannin extract are enhanced in combination with other polyphenols as found in pomegranate juice. J Nutr Biochem 2005 Jun; 16(6):360-67.

12. Sartippour MR et al. Ellagitannin-rich pomegranate extract inhibits angiogenesis in prostate cancer in vitro and in vivo. Intl J Oncol 2008; 32:475-80.

13. Pantuck AJ, et al. Phase II study of pomegranate juice for men with rising prostate-specific antigen following surgery or radiation for prostate cancer. Clin Cancer Res 2006; 12:4018-26.

14. Zhang Q, Radisavljevic ZM, Siroky MB, Azadzoi KM. Dietary antioxidants improve arteriogenic erectile dysfunction. Int J Androl. 2011 Jun;34(3):225-35. doi: 10.1111/j.1365-2605.2010.01083.x.

15. Schwarz S, Obermüller-Jevic UC, Hellmis E, Koch W, Jacobi G, Biesalski HK. Lycopene inhibits disease progression in patients with benign prostate hyperplasia. J Nutr. 2008 Jan;138(1):49-53.

16. Ziglioli F et al. Vanilloid-mediated apoptosis in prostate cancer cells through a TRPV-1 dependent and a TRPV-1-independent mechanism. Acta Biomed 2009 Apr; 80(1): 13-20.

17. Athanasiou A et al. Vanilloid receptor agonists and antagonists are mitochondrial inhibitors: how vanilloids cause non-vanilloid receptor mediated cell death. Biochem Biophys Res Commun 2007 Mar 2; 354(1): 50-55.

Prostate Treatment Can Cause Sex Problems

Erectile dysfunction can last 15 years or more

When men hear the words "prostate cancer" they often rush into treatment so fast they never even consider the side effects.

But there are side effects — life-altering and even life-ruining side effects, including sex problems that can last for years or even for the rest of your life.

In one new study, men who were treated for early stage prostate tumors suffered from lingering sex problems for years afterwards. Not just some of them, but nearly all of them.

And not just for a few years.

The study tracked 1,655 men between the ages of 55 and 74 at the start of the study, and 87 percent of the ones who had prostate surgery were suffering from sex problems a full 15 years later.

The numbers for men treated with radiation were even worse: 94 percent of them were battling sexual dysfunction 15 years later.

Now, it goes without saying that any large group of men in their 70s and 80s will include some guys with sex problems– but we know from other studies that it should be roughly half of them… not practically everyone.

And that wasn't the only problem that lingered through the years.

Eighteen percent of the men who had surgery and 9 percent of the ones who had radiation were battling urinary incontinence 15 years later, while 5 percent of the men who had surgery and 16 percent of those who underwent radiation were experiencing bowel issues.

Of course, if prostate surgery and radiation saved lives, you can argue that maybe it's worth all those risks and more.

But we know from other studies that many — maybe all — of these men would have survived even without radical treatment options such as surgery and radiation.

In one study I told you about last summer, men with prostate cancer were assigned to either surgery or no treatment at all. A decade later, there were no significant differences in the death rates.

That's because in many cases, prostate tumors grow so slowly that they simply do not pose a threat during a normal human lifespan — especially the early-stage tumors like the ones treated in the new study.

Instead of rushing into surgery, many senior men with prostate cancer would do well with an approach called watchful waiting. It's exactly what it sounds like: Keep an eye on the tumor, but don't treat it unless it starts to grow.

One way to help make sure that tumor stays small and worry-free is to not worry about it yourself — because stress alone can actually help feed many tumors, especially prostate tumors.

In experiments on mice that had human prostate cancer cells implanted in them, researchers found they were able to wipe out the cancer cells with medication when the mice were left unstressed.

But when the mice were stressed, the drug didn't work at all — and the cells kept growing.

So watch the tumor and watch your stress — and don't forget to include some prostate-friendly nutrients in your regimen, including vitamin D, turmeric, and selenium.

If surgery is indicated consult with a surgeon who has a lot of experience using robotic prostate surgery to reduce your risk of complications.

Work closely with a holistic physician on a nutritional approach that's right for you.

Dietary Changes Can Slash
Risk of Prostate Cancer

Simple steps to reduce prostate risk

The best offense is a good defense — that's as true in your body as it is in sports.

It's especially true when it comes to fighting cancer, because the best way to beat the disease is to make sure you never get it in the first place.

Unlike sports, you don't need to sign an expensive free agent to improve your own defensive line. All you need to do is make a few changes to your diet and you can not only reduce the overall risk of prostate cancer, but also help make sure you avoid the deadliest forms of the disease.

First, boost your fiber intake. More fiber will slash your risk of the most aggressive form of prostate cancer by as much as 80 percent, according to one new study.

Next, ditch the junky refined carbohydrates most people eat these days and replace them with complex carbs, while eating a sensible amount of protein and fat. These changes will send your risk of prostate cancer plunging by between 60 and 70 percent, according to the study presented at the American Urological Association's annual meeting.

And third, give up milk — because a second new study finds men who drink milk have not only a higher risk of prostate cancer, but a higher risk of the most aggressive form of the disease.

We weren't designed to drink cow's milk anyway. If you want something healthy, refreshing and milk-like, switch to nut milks instead.

A sensible diet will of course help reduce your risk of obesity and ensure you avoid metabolic syndrome — or a collection of risk factors that include obesity, elevated blood sugar, high triglycerides, low HDL (aka "good") cholesterol and high blood pressure.

The more of these risk factors you have, the higher your risk of prostate cancer climbs. If you've got two of them, your risk of a high-grade prostate tumor jumps by 35 percent.

And if you've got three or four, that risk nearly doubles.

Of course, prostate cancer isn't the only risk of metabolic syndrome. If the cancer doesn't scare you, maybe diabetes, heart disease and an early death will — because metabolic syndrome will increase your risk of all that and more.

It doesn't take much to avoid it all. Just eat a little better, and your defense against disease will improve — no high-priced free agents necessary.

CHAPTER 6

How to Prevent Colon Cancer

Colonoscopies save lives:
A cancer screening that really works

The only thing better than a cancer cure is a cancer that doesn't need to be cured in the first place because your doctor caught it early.

Docs use that line to push all kinds of cancer screenings, including procedures you don't need and some that may end up doing you more harm than good. But there's one you *do* need — one very mainstream cancer screening that, surprisingly, works as advertised – colonoscopies.

Now, I know the power of that word. When I use it in person in my clinic, it has the power to get patients looking for the nearest exit.

By email, who knows… maybe you've already hit the "delete" button.

I hope you haven't, because two new studies confirm that this simple, safe and (believe it or not) painless procedure has the power to save your life. Get scoped, and your risk of death from colon cancer will plunge by 56 percent.

That makes colonoscopies one of the most effective techniques for beating any cancer of any kind.

Other colon screenings can also help, but not nearly as much. A fecal occult test will cut your risk by a third, while sigmoidoscopy — which uses a shorter tube and looks at only part of the colon — can reduce the risk by 40 percent.

The study didn't look at "virtual" colonoscopies, but other studies

Fast colonoscopies miss more precancerous cells
Six minutes that can save your life

Three minutes versus six minutes. It may not sound like much of a difference at all — either way, it's just a few minutes. But when it comes to colonoscopy, the difference between three minutes and six minutes could be the difference between life and death.

Six minutes is considered the gold standard for "withdrawal time," or the amount of time it takes to pull the scope from the colon. That's when the doc looks for precancerous cells and growths, and removes polyps.

But some docs cut corners — maybe they're overconfident, or maybe they just have lunch reservations — and pull out faster, flying through the procedure in just three minutes.

Well, you know what happens when you hurry, right? You miss things — and docs who speed through the procedure in three minutes miss more than twice as many polyps and nearly double the amount of precancerous cells and adenomas in the colon as docs who take the full six minutes, according to new research.

Now, I don't think you need a study to know you want a doctor willing to put a few extra minutes into your colon and locating precancerous cells.

The problem, of course, is that most people are under anesthesia during a colonoscopy — so you don't really know how much time your doc spent hunting for polyps.

That means you have to do a little homework before choosing a doctor — and don't be afraid to ask him some questions, like how much time he typically spends looking for polyps. Most doctors — good ones anyway — can tell you, probably down to the second.

And along with choosing the right doctor, make sure you choose the right procedure — a real colonoscopy instead of a virtual one. I know virtual procedures may sound better, but patients actually report more comfort and less pain during and after a real colonoscopy. Just as important, with virtual colonoscopy you're exposed to unnecessary radiation and if a polyp or growth is formed you will still need a regular colonoscopy anyway.

There's a lot of debate over many cancer screenings these days and which ones may or may not be necessary. But there's not much debate over colonoscopy. It's one of those areas where both mainstream and holistic physicians agree: These precancerous cells screenings save lives, so be sure to get one yourself.

have shown it's not as effective as the real deal (in addition to exposing you to far too much radiation).

But most people don't choose a virtual colonoscopy or a sigmoidoscopy because they think it's more effective. They choose these procedures because they think they're more comfortable — and that's just not true.

In real colonoscopies, you're put under general anesthesia. As a result, you don't feel a thing beyond a little grogginess when you wake up.

During a sigmoidoscopy and virtual colonoscopy, on the other hand, you'll be wide awake — and you'll feel plenty, which is why patients who've had real and virtual procedures prefer traditional colonoscopy by nearly every measure.

So skip the shortcuts and get yourself a real colonoscopy. Schedule it early, as studies show doctors are sharper and detect more polyps during morning procedures.

Since you can't eat until it's over, getting it out of the way early also means you don't have to deal with hunger pangs all day.

Patients Say Real Colonoscopy Has Less Pain than Virtual Ones

Patients prefer real colonoscopies to virtual ones

When a patient hears the word "colonoscopy," he starts looking for the door — and that view of his rear end fleeing the room is usually about as close as a doctor will get to examining his backside.

People are just terrified by the procedure, and for no good reason. It's relatively painless and highly effective. It not only detects the growths that cause colon cancer, but also removes them.

No growths, no cancer — and that's why people who get regular colonoscopies simply don't die of the disease.

But most patients don't even want to talk about it. It sounds painful… uncomfortable… and for some people, even a conversation about "butt health" can be a little embarrassing.

Some doctors have been pushing the less invasive "virtual" colonoscopy because patients seem to think it's a lot more comfortable — but a new study shows that's not the case.

Researchers gave both procedures to 90 patients between the ages of 19 and 65 years old, and then asked them which one they preferred.

Turns out, the real deal beat "virtual" colonoscopy in just about every measure. Patients say they had less anxiety, less pain, and even liked the exam rooms better when they got the real colonoscopies.

That might sound a little counterintuitive, but remember that patients who get a real colonoscopy get sedated.

Patients who get the virtual procedure do not.

As a result, patients who get a real colonoscopy don't feel a thing (some even fall asleep). Patients who get a "virtual" one do — and while the "virtual" name might make it sound like a procedure that takes place on a computer screen instead of in your body, that's not quite the case.

There's no scope in a virtual colonoscopy (unless polyps are detected), but a thin tube is put into the rectum so air can be pumped in. This inflates the colon and makes it easier to see.

It doesn't hurt. But patients say it's not the most comfortable thing in the world, either — and that's reflected in the 69 percent of patients in the survey who said the real colonoscopy had less pain.

In addition, a full 77 percent said they would choose the real colonoscopy over the virtual procedure in the future.

In other words, the real procedure isn't nearly as bad as most people fear. But there are other reasons why I prefer the real deal to the virtual ones.

First, virtual colonoscopy a relatively new technology and there are still question marks over its effectiveness.

Second, and more importantly, it uses a CT scan — and CT scans rely on radiation. It seems a little backwards to me to use cancer-causing radiation to detect and treat cancer... but then again, a lot of the cancer screenings and treatments out there are backwards.

Third, if you have polyps or a suspicious-looking lesion, you'll need to get another regular colonoscopy to biopsy the lesion — leading to the very procedure you were trying to avoid in the first place.

So skip the gimmicks, and along with "virtual" colonoscopies that means avoiding the less thorough (and cheaper) sigmoidoscopy. And definitely stay away from the up-and-coming procedure, the "laxative-free" colonoscopy — because it's really just another version of the virtual colonoscopy.

Real colonoscopies are proven, and they work — and they represent one of the best examples of mainstream medicine getting it right.

I don't see any reason to mess with success.

PS: If you have diabetes, be sure to start screening earlier — at 40 instead of 50. New research shows that diabetics in their 40s have the same risk of precancerous colon growths as non-diabetics in their 50s. It's as if the disease ages the colon by an entire decade.

CHAPTER 7

How to Prevent Breast Cancer

Breast Cancer Screening Effective?

Mammograms not so effective after all?

Listen to the advice dished out on TV every day, and you might think mammograms are the best and only form of breast cancer screening. But they're not the only way, of course, and they're certainly far from perfect when it comes to screening for this deadly cancer.

Now, new research shows just how far from perfect they really are: They're often no better than regular breast exams.

In the study, some 90,000 Canadian women were either given regular mammograms or told to avoid the breast cancer screening completely and get regular breast exams from a trained nurse instead.

Over 25 years, both groups had the exact same rate of death from breast cancer.

So far, that's a tie — but if you're thinking "better safe than sorry" and planning to schedule a mammogram anyway, think again.

While both groups had the same death rate, the treatment rates were vastly different, with women given mammograms far more likely to get treated for breast cancer.

Since the extra treatments and breast cancer screenings didn't add up to extra lives saved, that means they were for nothing — and these weren't just instances, either. The numbers add up to more than 1 in 5 cancer treatments being entirely unnecessary.

And if you include treatment for ductal carcinoma in situ (which usually results in a mastectomy), that number jumps to one in three.

There are other ways to have a breast cancer screening that allow doctors to get a clearer view of the breast and make more informed decisions about which tumors should be treated and which are best left alone.

I recommend ultrasound, MRIs or thermography.

The method that works best for you may depend on your risk factors for the disease such as family history, the density of your breast and more.

And of you have cancer, remember you have options — including time-tested cures that can be found hidden in the pages of the Bible (if you know where to look).

Lifestyle Tips for Preventing Breast Cancer

Lower risk factors for breast cancer
Two habits that will boost your risk factors for breast cancer

Breast cancer kills more than 40,000 American women a year. After lung cancer, it's the deadliest cancer in women — but there are two steps you can take right now that can help ensure you don't become part of this grim statistic.

And you can take both steps at the same time, because they're both related to what you eat.

Diet of course plays a major role in cancer risk for men and women alike, and two new studies confirm that both what you eat and how much you weigh can dramatically influence your risk factors breast cancer.

And if you eat a lot of unhealthy saturated fats, your risk is already far higher than it should be.

Women who eat the most saturated fat are 30 percent more likely to get three of the most common forms of breast cancer: estrogen receptor-positive (ER-positive), progesterone receptor-positive (PR-positive) and HER2-negative breast cancers.

In the study, women who ate the most saturated fats took in about 48 grams a day.

That's a lot of saturated fat — roughly triple the recommended daily limits — but sadly, too many women are eating that much or more each day.

Most of them get these fats from packaged foods, fast food and snack cakes — and along with increasing the risk of cancer, these unhealthy foods can also wreak havoc on your arteries and damage your heart.

And of course, it's a diet that's almost guaranteed to cause another one the major risk factors for breast cancer: obesity.

I'm sure you've heard about the so-called breast cancer gene, which increases the risk of the disease in some women. It's true. In a second new study, the gene was found to boost the risk of the disease by 70 percent.

But if you have that genetic marker and you're overweight or obese, that risk climbs by 210 percent.

In other words, your weight is a much bigger risk factor than your genes, according to the study presented at a recent meeting of the American Association for Cancer Research.

The answer here is simple: Lose weight and eat better, and your cancer risk will plunge even if you're genetically predisposed to the disease. You'll also enjoy overall good health, and a lower risk of heart attack, stroke and more.

I recommend a Mediterranean diet naturally low in saturated fats and loaded with many of the delicious foods you already love.

Walking can slash breast cancer risk factors
Breast cancer survivors: Go for a walk

Surviving breast cancer and beating breast cancer risk factors is winning a battle — but the war continues for the rest of your life.

And if you've survived this cancer yourself, you know better than anyone else that beating this disease is about more than just going through treatment and coming out the other side with a pulse.

It's about making sure the cancer doesn't rise again like a movie villain everyone thought was dead.

Now, new research on breast cancer risk factors shows an easy way you can almost guarantee your breast cancer never returns to hurt you — and it's not a drug, a food or even a vitamin.

It's a daily jog or run.

All it takes is 2.25 miles a day, or 9 laps around the track at the local high school — a distance most moderately healthy people can cover in less than half an hour.

But it really doesn't matter how long it takes. All that matters is that you do it, because breast cancer survivors who jog or run 2.25 miles a day cut their risk of death from the disease by 95 percent.

Now, I realize the last thing you feel like doing right after a cancer battle is going out for a run.

Some days, you're happy if you can just stand up.

But this doesn't mean training for a marathon the moment your treatment ends.

Start slow, and work you way up — because the study in the *International Journal of Cancer* finds that every mile you walk per day or every two-thirds of a mile that you run will cut your risk of death from breast cancer by 25 percent.

As you get better at it (and you will), pick up the pace. Work your way up from a walk to a jog to a run, because the study finds that running is 40 percent more effective than walking at cutting your death risk.

Eventually, you'll be able to do the 2.25 miles and barely break a sweat.

Along with being active every day, there are other steps you can take to cut your breast cancer risk factors recurrence and lowering your risk of death.

First, eat more cruciferous vegetables — including broccoli, Brussels sprouts and cabbage.

These naturally detoxifying vegetables can cut your risk of a breast cancer recurrence by 35 percent and slash your risk of death from the disease by 62 percent.

Second, eat more fresh fruits and vegetables overall. The more you eat, the lower your risk — with 10 servings a day reducing your risk of recurrence by nearly a third.

Fruits and vegetables rich in carotenoids are especially effective against breast cancer risk factors, so load up on carrots, spinach, kale, papaya, guava, tomatoes, sweet potatoes and collard greens.

Third, take a quality multivitamin with minerals each day. Breast cancer survivors who take this simple step are nearly a third less likely to suffer from a recurrence and less likely to die of the disease.

Finally, work closely with a holistic doctor who can help identify other nutrients you may need to help fight cancer, prevent a recurrence and support your overall health and wellbeing.

Carotenoids can help you avoid breast cancer
Vegetables can slash breast risk

If there are two words that can scare a woman more than "breast cancer" I can't think of them.

And where there's fear, there's money to be made — so every day, doctors exploit cancer fears to push women into unnecessary treatments when they should be focusing on prevention with a diet and full of vegetables with carotenoids. In some extreme cases, women who don't even have cancer take toxic drugs or undergo disfiguring surgeries in the hopes of preventing it.

It's crazy. And irresponsible, too — especially since you don't have to resort to extremes to lower your cancer risk. Just resort to better eating — including the nutrient-rich super-foods that will give your body the power to fight cancer on its own.

Start with the carotenoids found in carrots, spinach, kale, and more, as one new analysis finds that women who eat the most of these super-foods have the lowest risk of breast cancer.

Harvard University researchers looked at 80 percent of all the published data on carotenoids and breast cancer and found that women with the highest blood levels of these nutrients were between 15 percent and 20 percent less likely to get breast cancer than women with lower blood levels.

Since different fruits and vegetables provide different types of carotenoids, be sure to vary your diet — and along with the carrots, spinach, and kale I mentioned earlier, enjoy papaya, guava, tomatoes, sweet potatoes, and collard greens.

And as long as you're getting some variety, don't stop with carotenoid-rich vegetables. Also be sure to enjoy some cruciferous vegetables such as broccoli, cabbage, and — once again — kale, since they can also help slash the risk of breast cancer.

This isn't just good advice for avoiding breast cancer. A diet rich in fruits and vegetables can also help you survive the disease if you do get it, minimize the damage of mainstream treatments, and keep it from coming back.

In one recent study, breast cancer survivors who had 10 or more servings of fruits and vegetables a day cut the risk of a recurrence by nearly a third.

So whether you've already had the disease, or just want to make sure you don't get it, don't go extreme. Just go for more veggies.

Calcium channel blockers boost breast cancer risk
BP meds in new cancer link

Ladies, I've got some very bad news about some very common drugs — medications used so frequently that they're among the top 10 most widely used drugs in the nation.

They're so common that you almost certainly know someone who's taking them. You might even be using them yourself.

They're the calcium channel blockers often given to patients with high blood pressure — and they're popular for a reason: They deliver.

They're very effective at bringing BP levels down.

But safety is another story, especially for women — because new research finds calcium channel blockers can increase your risk of breast cancer, especially if you take them over the long term.

Use them for 10 years or more, and your risk of ductal breast cancer can shoot up by 2.4 times, while your risk of lobular breast cancer can jump by 2.6 times.

It doesn't matter if you take the long-acting drugs or the short-acting versions. Either way, the risks are the same, according to the study in the *Journal of the American Medical Association*.

Other calcium channel blockers don't seem to increase the risk, according to the study, and that might make it tempting to switch from one drug to another.

But why bother?

They all come with risks — different risks, but risks just the same, and the real answer here isn't to trade one set of those risks for another.

It's to find a way off the meds completely. And when it comes to blood pressure meds, I'm here to tell you that there's a real way off.

I know there is, because I help my own patients with natural BP control all the time. And today, I'm going to help you.

Start with the basic lifestyle changes you know you should be making anyway. Eat better, lose some weight and be more active. In most cases, those three steps alone will bring your BP levels down.

But if your levels don't fall — or if they don't fall far enough — you still have options, including natural remedies such as magnesium, fish oil and coenzyme Q10.

A holistic physician can help find the approach that'll work best for you.

Red meat increases breast cancer risk
Foods that can cause breast cancer

Your diet and your cancer risk are directly related, and that's a fact no matter who you are. But if you're a woman and you're at all concerned about your breast cancer risk (as you should be) there's one food you need to limit right now.

But unfortunately, it's one of the foods we eat most often in the United States.

It's red meat. And while you can enjoy it on occasion and in moderation, eating too much — and eating it too often — can increase your risk of breast cancer, according to new research.

A serving and a half a day will cause your risk to jump by 22 percent, and every serving on top of that will boost your risk by another 13 percent when compared to women who eat it once a week or less.

And remember, a "serving" isn't a "helping."

When many people eat red meat, they eat two servings or more at a time, making it frighteningly easy to reach dangerous levels without even realizing it.

But I'm not here to take the dinner off your plate.

While you should limit your red meat intake, there are other delicious foods that can do just the opposite, slashing your risk of breast cancer. Replacing that red meat with poultry, for example, will send your breast cancer risk plunging by 17 percent.

And if you're past menopause, eating more poultry will cause your risk to plunge by as much as 24 percent, according to the study of nearly 89,000 women tracked for up to 20 years.

Other foods that can help reduce your breast cancer risk include fish, legumes and nuts. Any combination of poultry, fish, legumes and nuts in place of red meat will reduce the risk of breast cancer by 14 percent, according to the study in *BMJ*.

This is great diet advice for anyone to follow, since these same foods can help cut your risk of everything from diabetes to stroke to heart disease. But if you're a woman and you're at risk for breast cancer, it could mean the difference between life and death.

Lifestyle Tips After
Breast Cancer Diagnosis

Breast cancer drugs don't save lives
Cancer drug isn't as good as advertised

On the surface, it must seem like a miracle pill: Cancer drugs that can slash the risk of breast cancer in women with the highest risk of the disease by nearly 40 percent.

New research confirms that estrogen-blocking cancer drugs such as tamoxifen really do deliver in that regard — and the study is already being used to push these meds on millions of new patients, including "high-risk" but otherwise healthy women with no sign of the disease at all.

But don't swallow that pill just yet — because there's more to this story.

While the headlines are focusing on that one finding — the lower risk of cancer — the study in *The Lancet* also finds that the breast cancer drugs have no impact at all on the disease's survival rates.

In other words, they haven't saved a single life despite that drop in cancer risk.

How could that be? Simple: The breast cancer drugs are likely preventing only the harmless tumors that are usually best left alone with a "watch and wait" approach.

Now, I understand why some women might know all that and choose to take the drug anyway. No one wants the stress and angst of a cancer diagnosis, even if the disease itself is survivable.

But the breast cancer drugs come with risks of their own, starting with the fact that they could actually increase the risk of other cancers — including cancer of the uterus. The potential risk is so great that the American Cancer Society lists tamoxifen as a known carcinogen.

In addition, there's evidence the drug may increase the risk of blood clots and stroke.

And since the drugs work by blocking estrogen, you also could face all the risks that come with shrinking hormone levels — including night sweats, hot flashes, skin conditions, and more.

There are better and safer ways to slash your risk of cancer without upsetting your hormone balance, and I've told you about a few of them recently.

Start by adding some natural detoxifiers to your menu, especially cruciferous vegetables such as broccoli, cabbage, and kale. These natural cancer-fighters can decrease the risk of dying of breast cancer by more than a third.

In addition, the carotenoids found in some cruciferous vegetables as well as carrots and other veggies can reduce your risk of breast cancer by as much as 20 percent, according to Harvard University research. These vegetables don't come with any risks, only benefits and great taste.

The cancer-busting diet you can start today

What do tumors and bellies have in common? They both get bigger on a high-carb diet.

A new study on mice finds that a low-carb diet can slow, stop, and even prevent cancer.

Researchers from the British Columbia Cancer Research Center in Canada injected different types of tumors into mice and then put them onto either a typical Western diet (55 percent carbs, 23 percent protein, and 22 percent fat), or a low-carb diet (15 percent carbs, 25 percent fat, and 60 percent protein).

Even though the diets had the same number of calories, the carb-happy mice put on more weight. Even more alarmingly, their tumors grew consistently faster — as if they were powered by carbs.

The researchers also carried out a similar experiment on mice predisposed to breast cancer and found that nearly half of those on the Western diet got the disease in their first year... versus none among the low-carb mice.

Over the longer term, only 30 percent of the low-carb mice developed the disease before they died, versus 70 percent of rodents on the high-carb diet.

The researchers wrote in Cancer Research that although the rodents had a two-year life expectancy, only one of the mice in the high-carb group reached it — while half the mice in the low-carb group reached or beat that expiration date.

Obviously, it's a study on mice — not people. But the researchers say the connection was so strong that it seems highly likely that it would apply to humans as well.

And that means if you're not on a low-carb diet yet, you might want to get started on one ASAP.

In addition to lowering your risk for cancer and causing tumors to starve, a high-protein diet low in sugar and other carbohydrates can slash your risk for diabetes, heart disease and more.

And if you've heard that a low-carb diet is bad for your arteries, you heard wrong: A recent study found no difference in vascular health between low-carb dieters and those who tried the low-fat approach.

Another mainstream myth bites the dust!

If all those health benefits of a low-carb diet aren't enough, consider this: It's also the fastest way to lose weight… and the surest way to keep it off for good.

Vegetables with the power to beat cancer
There's something about broccoli

It has the power to stop breast tumors from growing… and you can find it in your local supermarket for less than $2 a pound.

Broccoli and other cruciferous vegetables have long been recognized by science for their cancer-fighting powers, especially when it comes to breast cancers, but researchers have taken it to the next level by isolating the main compound believed to help put the brakes on tumors.

It's called glucoraphanin, and on its own it doesn't do much.

But when the vegetable is damaged — like when you eat it — it gets converted into a molecule called sulforaphane that can boost antioxidant levels in the body and even fight off the enzyme that allows tumors to grow.

There's even evidence it can stimulate the production of other cancer-fighting enzymes in the body.

Put it all together, and you can see why one recent study found that women who eat the most cruciferous vegetables are 62 percent less likely to die of breast cancer and 35 percent less likely to have a recurrence than those who eat the least.

And that's also why there's a race to turn broccoli into a cancer-fighting "drug."

In two promising clinical trials under way right now, researchers are giving different levels of sulforaphane to cancer patients, and you can bet I'll keep you posted on the progress of those studies.

But in the meantime, you can get the same levels of this molecule — and more — without making too many changes to your diet. In fact, researchers say just three or four servings of cruciferous veggies a week should be enough to do the trick.

The best sources of glucoraphanin are broccoli sprouts, especially young sprouts, but you'll also find it in regular broccoli, cabbage, and Brussels sprouts. Cooked right, they're also delicious.

But if they can beat cancer, I'd say they're worth eating even if you don't love the taste.

Broccoli beats breast cancer

I recommend cruciferous vegetables for detoxification so often that I'm sure some of my patients think I own stock in a broccoli farm.

In the interest of full disclosure, I should point out that I don't

— but if I ever decided to get into the agricultural business, I'd grow cruciferous vegetables like broccoli, cabbage, and kale.

They're that good.

When you detox with these vegetables, you not only rid your body of toxins, you also give it the power to fight cancer — and the latest research shows why women in particular should make sure they boost their intake of these veggies.

In a new study out of China, researchers found that breast cancer patients who had the highest intake of cruciferous vegetables were 62 percent less likely to die of the disease and 35 percent less likely to have a recurrence when compared to those who ate the least.

The study of nearly 5,000 women between the ages of 20 and 75 even found that those who ate the most of these vegetables had a lower risk of death from all causes.

A coincidence? I don't think so — because cruciferous vegetables are rich in powerful glucosinolates, which break down to form isothiocyanates. You don't have to memorize either tongue-twisting word, just remember this: isothiocyanates can fight tumors and even cause cancer cells to commit suicide.

They're so powerful that the drug industry is trying to develop cancer meds based on isothiocyanates — but why wait for their synthetic version when you can get your own natural daily dose the delicious way?

Our most common cruciferous vegetables include broccoli, cauliflower, and Brussels sprouts, but it's worth noting that the women in this study ate a more typical Chinese diet — and their most common cruciferous vegetables include bok choy, Chinese cabbage, and turnips.

More importantly, they also eat a lot more of these vegetables overall — so if you want to take advantage of those cancer-fighting properties yourself, make sure you increase your own intake.

And if you haven't tried bok choy, you've been missing out.

Essential vitamins can prevent death from breast cancer
One of these every day can beat breast cancer

Breast cancer awareness month just ended, and I've seen plenty of pink ribbons and I've heard all the usual propaganda about mammograms — but I haven't heard a single word about what just might be the most powerful weapon against this disease yet.

It's simple, safe and inexpensive. And if you've been taking my advice, it's something that's already part of your life.

It's your multivitamin — specifically a multi with minerals, as new research finds these daily essential vitamins can slash your risk of death from breast cancer by nearly a third.

There's not much else out there with a benefit that big, ladies — but like all good things, essential vitamins comes with a catch: You have to start now, because the study finds the life-saving benefits go to women already taking a multi when they're diagnosed.

That suggests to me that the nutrients and minerals in the essential vitamins help your body fight the tumor early on, making sure it stays treatable and survivable instead of turning aggressive and deadly.

Now, any time a study finds big benefits for multivitamins, mainstream experts line up to dismiss it. They never attack the studies, because the studies are sound.

No, instead they attack the essential vitamins — claiming most people don't need them because you can get all your nutrients from diet alone.

And that just ignores reality.

It's difficult, and maybe even close to impossible, to get absolutely everything you need, every day, from diet alone. Even a healthy diet loaded with nutrient-rich foods can fall short in some key areas.

A multi is there to fill in the blanks and make sure you're covered, day in and day out — and along with helping to fight breast cancer, studies have found plenty of other benefits.

Ladies, a multivitamin can help lift your mood and reduce your risk of stress, anxiety, fatigue and more, according to a study I told you about earlier this year.

Men, don't feel left out — because multivitamins can slash your risk of all non-prostate cancers by 12 percent, according to another recent study. And in children, multivitamins can help during the most critical stages of development.

But whatever you do, don't go for the low-price vitamins in the supermarket discount bin. Choose a quality multi from a maker you trust.

Yes, they cost a little more — but it's the best way to make sure you get the right amounts of the nutrients you need most in the forms your body can use best.

Breast cancer patients need exercise

What every breast cancer patient needs to do

Cancer is exhausting.

If the disease itself doesn't sap you of all your strength, energy and will, the mainstream treatments for it will rob you of whatever's left.

As a result, many cancer patients don't get much activity at all.

I can't say I blame them. I know how difficult it is. But I'm going to ask you to reach down deep inside and find the energy to get regular activity, especially if you're locked in a battle with breast cancer — because exercise isn't optional at this point.

It's critical to your survival.

Exercise is proven to not only prevent breast cancer, but also ensure that you don't die of it if you do get the disease. But a new study finds that most breast cancer patients rarely get anything close to the level of activity they truly need.

Overall, 59 percent of breast cancer survivors reduce their levels of physical activity after their diagnosis. Even worse, 65 percent fail to meet guidelines, which recommend at least 150 minutes of moderate activity or 75 minutes of vigorous activity per week.

That means just 35 percent of breast cancer patients and survivors get the exercise they need to survive and thrive.

And that's a tragic mistake.

If you're a breast cancer survivor, even moderate activity — a brisk, 30-minute walk several times a week — will slash your risk of dying from the disease by 40 percent, according to one study.

And the more activity you get, the more that survival benefit grows.

Exercise is also an effective way of fighting off the side effects of cancer treatments.

And if that's not enough motivation to get you moving, exercise is also proven to lift the mood, ward off depression and enhance the overall quality of life in breast cancer survivors.

But don't wait for disease to strike to get moving. If you don't have breast cancer, start exercising now — because other studies have shown that regular movement can cut your risk of getting the disease by as much as a fifth.

Simple Wheat Germ Extract Revealed to Be a **Powerful Cancer Fighter**

There's a natural and powerful anti-cancer therapy hiding in a common food that's practically unknown to almost every oncologist in North America. Yet, if you travel to a country such as Hungary you will find that it's an accepted therapy by cancer specialists. I'm talking about fermented wheat germ extract (FWGE). This special extract is different than the wheat germ oil you'll find on the shelves of your local health food store.

FWGE was developed by Dr. Mate Hidvegi, a Hungarian chemist, in the 1990s. He was following up on the work of Dr. Albert Szent Gyorgyi who received the Nobel Prize in Medicine in 1937 for the discovery of vitamin C and the life-sustaining processes of cellular metabolism. Dr. Gyorgyi theorized that substances known as benzoquinones, (also known as DMBQ's), play a critical role in glucose metabolism. Before completing his work in this area he died in 1986.

Dr. Mate Hidvégi followed up on this research with a team of scientists. He developed a patented process of fermenting wheat germ with baker's yeast. The result was a well-researched natural substance with more than 100 studies described in over 20 peer-reviewed medical journals.

For example, it has been studied at UCLA, General Clinical Research Center and Clinical Nutrition Research Unit as well as The Scientific Program, NATO. Many of those studies explored its use for the complementary treatment of cancer.

How FWGE works

FWGE has unique actions in the body that make it a powerful assistant in the fight against cancer. You see cancer cells thrive on glucose, using the sugar for fuel. But fermented wheat germ blocks those cells from gobbling up the glucose. It accomplishes this by inhibiting an enzyme known as glucose-6-phosphate dehydrogenase (G6PDH) which is required for glucose metabolism. Studies show it can inhibit this enzyme by up to a stunning 95 percent.[1] Without a fuel supply the cancer cells are unable to grow and eventually they die.

But FWGE's anti-cancer actions don't stop there. Not by a long shot. In fact, the wheat germ hits cancer with not just one but two more cancer-killing punches. First, FWGE reduces the amount of a specific protein found on tumor cells. When this protein is curbed it gives the body's *own* cancer-killing immune cells the opening they need to attack the cancer cells more effectively. Second, FWGE completes the job by supercharging the activity of certain immune cells that target tumors.

There are likely a number of components of FWGE that gives it its unique anti-cancer properties, but the best studied is a group of chemicals called benzoquinones. (I mentioned them earlier.) Wheat germ naturally contains some benzoquinones and the fermentation process causes their levels to skyrocket. And the higher the benzoquinones levels are, the higher the anticancer potential of FWGE is.

Regular wheat germ extract doesn't have nearly the levels of benzoquinones that the fermented version has, and this is why the run-of-the-mill extracts don't have similar therapeutic activity. And, most importantly, *unlike* chemotherapy and radiation FWGE is able to accomplish its anti-cancer effects *without* doing any damage to healthy cells in the process.

Let's take a look at a couple of those over 100 studies on FWGE that I mentioned earlier. There are plenty to choose from, but let's focus on just a few of the human studies today. These studies show an overall improvement in survival, disease-free survival, and improved quality of life.

Kicking colorectal cancer

Hungarian researchers tested the effect of FWGE on sixty-six patients with colorectal cancer. The volunteers received FWGE supplementation for more than 6 months while 104 control patients received traditional anticancer therapies alone. By the end of the study 23 percent of the patients receiving conventional cancer treatments had their cancer spread. In sharp contrast, only eight percent of the FWGE patients saw their cancer spread.[2]

Melanoma meets its match

In one randomized clinical trial, patients with melanoma were given standard chemotherapy or chemotherapy plus FWGE for one year. After a seven-year follow up period, researchers found that patients who had taken FWGE were *half* as likely to die from melanoma during this time.[3]

Opting out of oral cancers

There's very little research available on natural products for cancers of the mouth and neck so I was pleased to uncover such positive research on FWGE. Researchers followed 22 patients with oral cancer who took FWGE and compared them with 21 patients not receiving FWGE. Those who took FWGE reduced the risk for cancer progression by a stunning 85 percent.[4]

In fact, FWGE's abilities to fight the spread of oral cancer are so impressive that when the Hungarian Association of Oral and Maxillofacial Surgeons reviewed the research they sung the fermented wheat germ's praises saying:

"For patients suffering from head and neck tumors—primarily malignant tumorous diseases of the oral cavity, the progression of the disease can be slowed significantly, the five-year survival rate increased considerably, the quality of life improved, and the oxidative stress on the patients reduced by the long-term application of the supplementary formula Avemar (FWGE). The Association considers the supportive treatment with the formula Avemar as an important part of the complex therapeutic protocols applied in stages II, III and IV of malignant tumorous diseases of the oral cavity."[5] I'd call that a ringing endorsement.

Curb chemo infections

One of the many risks with chemotherapy is the suppression of your white blood cells which fight infection. FWGE was found, in one study, to have the ability to head infections off at the pass in children and teenagers undergoing chemotherapy. When researchers followed 22 kids and teens who were being treated for different types of cancer they found that those who received FWGE had*significantly* fewer infections and fevers while receiving chemotherapy.[6]

Leave behind lung Cancer

At the Los Angeles Biomedical Research Institute at Harbor-UCLA Medical Center an open trial with 16 people with lung cancer who were receiving standard cancer therapy was supplemented with FWGE. Patient's symptoms and quality of life were monitored with a questionnaire. Researchers found a significant improvement in the overall state of health including a reduction in fatigue and pain, and an improvement in appetite and emotional state.[7]

Ban breast cancer

In 2004 Hungarian researchers put FWGE to the test against human breast cancer cells. When the fermented wheat germ was combined with the estrogen-blocking breast-cancer drug Tamoxifen it *increased* the rate of cancer cell death.[8]

Beat rheumatoid arthritis

Over the years I've told you about a number of natural substances that may help with the treatment of rheumatoid arthritis (RA) including collagen, MSM, fish oil, and turmeric. It looks like we might need to add FWGE to that list.

Interestingly, FWGE has been shown in preliminary studies to help people with their RA symptoms. In a year-long study patients with RA had a significant reduction in stiffness at their six- and 12-month follow up. Half of the participants were even able to reduce the amount of steroids they were taking.[9]

Dosage and usage details

In the morning before breakfast, I generally recommend taking one packet containing 8.5 to 9 g of FWGE daily mixed with eight ounces of cold water or any other beverage that contains less than 10 mg vitamin C per eight-ounce serving. Store the packets at room temperature or in the refrigerator. It's also available in tablets. The typical tablet dosage is 5 tabs twice a day on an empty stomach.

Side effects are very uncommon with FWGE. Some people occasionally have minor digestive upset and that can be relieved by dividing the dose in half twice daily.

Be sure to not take vitamin C supplements or beverages containing high amounts of vitamin C within two hours of ingesting FWGE. If you are pregnant, a nursing mother, have had an organ or tissue transplant, are suffering from bleeding gastrointestinal ulcers, malabsorption syndrome, gluten sensitive enterophaties (celiac sprue), fructose intolerance, or have hypersensitivity to gluten or wheat germ you should not use FWGE.

As I mentioned earlier, FWGE is very different from the wheat germ granules and wheat germ oil you may be familiar with. It comes in a powder and is sold in many health food stores, by health professionals, or online as a dietary supplement in the United States. I routinely prescribe it to patients who see me at my clinic for the complementary treatment of cancer because studies clearly show it improves cancer survival rates. Speak to a doctor skilled in natural medicine about adding this to your diet.

Sources:

1. Comin-Anduix B, Boros LG, Marin S, et al. Fermented wheat-germ extract inhibits glycolysis/pentose cycle enzymes and induces apoptosis through poly(ADP-ribose) polymerase activation in Jurkat T-cell leukemia tumor cells. J Biol Chem, 2002 Nov 29;277(48):46408-14.

2. Farkas E. Fermented wheat germ extract in the supportive therapy of colorectal cancer. Orv Hetil. 2005;146(37):1925-31.

3. Demidov LV, Manziuk LV, Kharkevitch GY, Pirogova NA, Artamonova EV, Adjuvant fermented wheat germ extract (Avemar) nutraceutical improves survival of high-risk skin melanoma patients: a randomized, pilot, phase II clinical study with a 7-year follow-up. Cancer Biother Radiopharm. 2008;23(4):477-82.

4. Barabás J, Németh Z. Recommendation of the Hungarian Society for Face, Mandible and Oral Surgery in the indication of supportive therapy with Avemar. Orv Hetil. 2006;147(35):1709-11.

5. J. Barabás, Zs. Németh. Recommendation of the Hungarian Association of Oral and Maxillofacial Surgeons (Magyar Arc-, Állcsont-és Szájsebészeti Társoság) in the indication of supportive therapy with Avemar. Hungarian Medical Journal. 2006 Volume 147, Issue 35, 1709–1711

6. Garami M, Schuler D, Babosa M, Borgulya G, Hauser P, Müller J, Paksy A, Szabó E, Hidvégi M, Fekete G. Fermented wheat germ extract reduces chemotherapy-induced febrile neutropenia in pediatric cancer patients, J Pediatr Hematol Oncol. 2004;26(10):631-5.

7. Boros LG, Nichelatti M, Shoenfeld Y. Fermented wheat germ extract (Avemar) in the treatment of cancer and autoimmune diseases. Ann N Y Acad Sci. 2005 Jun;1051:529-42.

8. Marcsek Z, Kocsis Z, Jakab M, Szende B, Tompa A. The efficacy of tamoxifen in estrogen receptor-positive breast cancer cells is enhanced by a medical nutriment. Cancer Biother Radiopharm. 2004 Dec;19(6):746-53.

9. Bálint G, Apáthy A, Gaál M, Telekes A, Resetár A, Blazsó G, Falkay G, Szende B, Paksy A, Ehrenfeld M, Shoenfeld Y, Hidvégi M., Effect of Avemar—a fermented wheat germ extract—on rheumatoid arthritis. Preliminary data, Clin Exp Rheumatol. 2006;24(3):325-8.)

Conquer Cancer Without Drugs

Conquer your cancer WITHOUT dangerous drugs — Target the root cause with this powerful all-natural solution

If you're waiting for conventional medicine to come up with a breakthrough cancer-preventing vaccine, or some other miracle method for definitively preventing or curing cancer I've got to warn you, you will be disappointed.

I remember just before attending medical school my father was diagnosed with cancer and was admitted to the hospital. He thought surgery and chemotherapy would magically solve his problems and he would be back to normal in no time. While he rarely saw a doctor of any kind, he was convinced conventional medicine had advanced so far that what was described as a "wimpy" cancer would be eradicated.

Having rarely missed a day of work in his life he died a few weeks later. It was then that I truly realized that, more often than not, conventional cancer therapy overpromises and under delivers. Many find that their experience with conventional cancer therapy leaves them feeling hopeless and undervalued. But the science of Integrative Oncology is changing all that, it's once again giving people hope.

Whether you realize it or not there's a worldwide war raging against cancer. According to The International Agency for Research on Cancer (IARC), the specialized cancer agency of the World Health Organization, there were 14.1 million new cases and 8.2 million cancer deaths in 2012. There are 32.6 million people (over the age of 15) alive today who have received a cancer diagnoses in the last five years.

Understanding chronic inflammation

In both conventional and holistic medicine we're taught that inflammation is related to most chronic diseases including cancer, cardiovascular disease, diabetes, Alzheimer's, and arthritis. But holistic doctors *also* acknowledge that inflammation, in of itself, is not a bad thing. Rather it's necessary for healing to take place, and a sign that your immune system is reacting to injury or infection. However, when your immune system goes on the blink... often called a dysfunctional or dysregulated immune system... and that inflammation becomes *chronic*, cell damage and abnormal cell replication kick in, setting the stage for cancer.

Instead of trying to mask inflammation, holistic doctors will always try to address the *root* causes. Root causes for inflammation can run the gamut, and can include:

- diet
- environmental toxins (pesticides, heavy metals, and industrial pollution)
- alcohol
- excess body weight
- excessive ultraviolet radiation
- electromagnetic pollution
- infections (viruses, bacteria, and fungi)
- pharmaceutical medications
- stress
- nutritional deficiencies
- lack of exercise
- genetics

Looking at that list one thing should seem pretty obvious. And that is that no single medication or medical procedure could possibly address *all* of the root causes of the chronic inflammation that fuels the fires of cancer. It's imperative that you address the root causes that you *do* have control over to avoid becoming a cancer statistic. Fortunately, genetically caused cancer is rare, and it isn't the main player for the vast majority of people. In fact, only 5% to 10% of cancers are inherited.[1]

In many (perhaps most) cases, cancer is entirely preventable and you can slash your risk for the disease by making changes in your diet, taking the proper supplements, getting regular exercise, managing your stress, detoxifying, avoiding toxins, refusing risky medications, and skipping questionable medical procedures. Even one of these changes can have a dramatic impact. For example, it's estimated that you can reduce your risk of cancer by up to 40% just by choosing to eat healthier foods.

This protein complex could be the key to conquering chronic diseases

One of the most exciting areas of research today focuses on identifying substances which will inhibit NF-κB (nuclear factor kappa-light-chain-enhancer of activated B cells). NF-κB is a protein complex that activates the genes and pathways that increase inflammation. Research has shown that the ongoing activation of NF-κB is linked with most cancers and most major diseases, for that matter. If we can learn how to inhibit or reduce the activity of NF-κB then we can potentially prevent or delay the onset of a number of chronic diseases, including cancer.

Drugs, of course, are already being developed to inhibit NF-κB, but since they're synthesized and unnatural a host of serious side effects will certainly come along with them. But there's *already* a natural substance that's showing terrific promise when it comes to inhibiting NF-κB. And instead of heading to a pharmacy to get it you can head straight for your spice rack.

Turmeric, the delicious and popular golden spice from Asia has been shown to have nearly miraculous biological activities when it comes to suppressing NF-κB, as well as impressive anti-cancer effects. At an oncology conference I recently attended, Bharat B. Aggarwal, Ph.D. (from The University of Texas, M.D. Anderson Cancer Center) spoke. Dr. Aggarwal is a world renowned expert on the medicinal uses of turmeric, and he pointed out that there have been well over 3,000 papers published on this incredible spice.[2] How many *drugs* can make a similar claim?

Tumeric's anti-cancer properties are impressive, to say the least. According to published research the spice can…

- suppress NF-κB and many other inflammatory compounds in the body
- stimulate apotoposis (cancer cell death)
- induce cancer cell proliferation
- inhibit blood supply to tumors
- inhibit the invasion of cancer
- inhibit the metastasis (spreading) of cancer
- reduce the side effects of chemotherapy
- reduce the cancerous compounds found in smokers

One of the qualities that makes turmeric so unique is its natural ability to target a variety of cancer-causing pathways including tumor suppressor genes, inflammatory biomarkers, growth factors signaling, transcription factors, apoptotic genes, oncoproteins, and protein kinases.

No prescription drug can match this simple spice's wide spectrum mechanism of action. But turmeric's abilities don't stop there. It also has the power to make chemotherapy and radiation therapies more effective, meaning that if you have chosen conventional treatments the spice could improve your response.

According to Dr. Aggarwal, there have been more than 65 human clinical trials—with more than 1000 volunteers—completed on turmeric so far. There are at least 35 more currently being performed on the spice. And research reveals a direct relationship between countries that consume a lot of spices like turmeric, and a significantly lower incidence of cancer. The United States consumes far less spices per capita than other large countries like China and India.

Interestingly, some nutrition-oriented doctors, including some oncologists, have begun administering turmeric extract as an intravenous therapy. This allows a higher concentration of the active compounds in turmeric to reach the cells of your body. Preliminary animal studies on intravenous turmeric have shown that the therapy may have anti-cancer effects.

Taking your turmeric

I recommend you liberally add turmeric to your favorite foods. It's a delicious addition to many meals. To avoid pesticides and heavy metal contamination make sure the turmeric you choose is organic. If you don't like the taste of turmeric, or you simply want to increase the amount of the spice you're getting, any health food store will carry turmeric capsules or tablets.

If you have cancer, discuss turmeric supplements with your doctor. I generally recommend a daily dose of 1500 to 3000 mg or higher. Studies haven't found any toxicity with this safe spice, even up to 10 grams a day! However, at higher doses, turmeric *can* cause occasional digestive upset. The spice also has a blood-thinning effect so make sure to check with your doctor first if you're already on any blood-thinning medications. Several good brands to consider include Nature's Way, Natural Factors, and New Chapter.

Statistically speaking

The American Cancer Society estimates that more than 1.6 million new cases of cancer were diagnosed in 2013. The most commonly diagnosed cancer in men is prostate cancer. For women it's breast cancer. Lung and colorectal cancers are the second and third most common cancers in both sexes. Men have a 1 in 2 lifetime probability of developing cancer, and for women it's 1 in 3.3.

Mastering turmeric terminology

Don't be confused when it comes to turmeric terminology. You'll often hear the term curcuminoids used when people speak about this spice. Curcuminoids is simply a group of active medicinal components found in turmeric. One of the better researched curcuminoids is curcumin.

Tell me about turmeric

Turmeric has a long history of being used as a food flavoring, a preservative, and a dye in Asian countries, especially India and China. The golden-yellow spice is the main component of most curry blends. In the United States turmeric is used to give mustard its yellow color. The supplement form of the spice is often used as a natural anti-inflammatory for conditions like arthritis, and more recently turmeric has been in the spotlight for its potential to fight cancer.

Citations

1. Ibid, http://www.cancer.org/cancer/cancercauses/geneticsandcancer/heredity-and-cancer

2. Bharat B. Aggarwal, Ph.D. Molecular Targets and Therapeutic Uses of Curcumin 3rd Annual Conference and Expo IV Therapies 2014 Integrative Oncology. January 25, 2014.

3. American Cancer Society website. Accessed March 16, 2014 at http://www.cancer.org/research/cancerfactsfigures/cancerfactsfigures/cancer-facts-figures-2013

The 5 Things You Must Know to Prevent Cancer Today

#1: Is Cancer on Tap in YOUR kitchen?

If you're a guy, I want you to put down that glass. Back slowly away from the sink. And whatever you do don't drink another sip of water until you answer one simple question for me.

Have you taken your birth control pills today?

Yes, I'm aware that it's an outrageous question. No man has ever *willingly* swallowed a birth control pill. But that's why what I'm about to tell you so disgraceful.

You may be shocked to learn that…

Your tap water may be laced with hormones

The fact is you could be swallowing birth control hormones with every sip you take of tap water. And with every swallow, those hormones could be sending your risk of prostate cancer climbing right through the roof.

It's not pleasant to think about, but it's reality. Leftovers from birth control pills, including synthetic estrogen and progestin, are *literally* being flushed down our toilets and contaminating our water supply. And unfortunately, those of us with a prostate gland are suffering the consequences since our prostates are particularly sensitive to hormones.

A recent study in the *British Medical Journal* (BMJ) took a deep look at the data we have available on prostate cancer. But, ironically, they didn't initially set out to learn anything about prostates at all. However, they just couldn't ignore the unintentional findings that their research was turning up.

Originally the team was researching how many women were using contraception, including birth control pills, intrauterine devices, condoms, or vaginal barriers. But they accidentally also uncovered a strong link between birth control pill use and cases of prostate cancer worldwide.

Making a rePEEt performance in your drinking glass

Birth control pills are in class of chemicals known as endocrine disturbing compounds. Other examples of endocrine disruptors include detergents, pesticides, cosmetics, and building materials. Whenever a woman on birth control pills pees, she literally releases hormone residues into the sewage system. And unfortunately water treatment facilities do not filter out these compounds, or even test to see if they are there. So they end up in our drinking water.

To be honest I've never been a fan of birth control pills as a form of contraception. They cause an imbalance in a woman's hormones and come with inherent risks such as breast cancer (yes, even the highly touted low-dose versions), weight gain, and blood clots. Now emerging evidence is showing the health hazards of these drugs extend to men as well. And I can only imagine what they're doing to our children.

Studies have already shown that contamination from these synthetic estrogens is causing infertility and deformities in animals. It only stands to reason that this should set off alarm bells about what they may be doing to humans as well. And this study in *BMJ* is not the first one to link them with health problems in humans. However, because the link was so significant, and seen worldwide, it <u>has</u> finally made more researchers sit up and take notice of the potential health hazards of these pills.

Protect yourself from prostate cancer

Prostate cancer is the most common male malignancy in the Western world. To lower your risks of becoming a victim you need to start protecting yourself against estrogen overload today. First, make sure you're drinking purified water. Water that's been run through a reverse-osmosis filter or distilled are both good options. And if you use a water bottle make sure it's bisphenol A free.

Next, eat one to two servings of cruciferous vegetables a day to help your body metabolize estrogen. Also be sure to get plenty of fiber into your diet. Regular bowel movements will help your body literally

SEVEN THINGS YOU NEVER KNEW...

1. Everything from antibiotics to Prozac have been found in the feathers of factory farm chickens. Skip the big supermarket brands and choose an organic bird instead.

2. Junk food can make you depressed. A new study out of Europe finds that a steady junk-food habit can boost your risk of depression by up to a whopping 51 percent!

3. The flavonoid rutin found in apples, onions, citrus fruits, asparagus, red wine and green tea can help prevent blood clots and reduce your risk of heart attack or stroke.

4. A positive attitude may literally ward off a heart attack. A recent Harvard analysis of more than 200 studies confirmed that an optimistic outlook could cut your risk of a first heart attack in half!

5. Despite what you may have heard eggs won't raise your cholesterol levels. But eating some at breakfast can help you feel less hungry and help you lose weight.

6. Besides the unhealthy fake butter you find in microwave popcorn, it can contain perfluorooctanoic acid (PFOA), a cancer-linked chemical used to manufacture the heat-resistant fluoropolymers used in some food packaging.

7. The curry spice turmeric may help you survive bypass surgery and even avoid a heart attack during your recovery.

expel harmful estrogens. And you should start using natural skin care products that are free of estrogenic parabens.

I often test the estrogen level of men. If the level is too high I put them on a detox program. This includes purified water, organic food, and ground flaxseeds. In addition I have them supplement their diet with phytonutrients such as indole 3 carbinol, diindolylmethane, and glutathione, which helps their livers rid their bodies of the extra estrogen.

Citation:

Margel D, Fleshner NE. Oral contraceptive use is associated with prostate cancer: an ecological study. BMJ Open 2011;1:e000311. doi:10.1136/bmjopen-2011-000311

#2: The Bitter Truth about Artificial Sweeteners and Cancer

You probably know aspartame by its brand names NutraSweet and Equal. The popular artificial sweetener is a staple on restaurant tables around the world. It adds the sweet taste to diet soda, instant tea, sugarless candy, and chewing gum. Heck, it's even dumped into over-the-counter cough syrups and liquid pain relievers to make them syrupy sweet.

Aspartame is popular because it tastes similar to sugar but adds no calories to foods. According to the Calorie Control Council, the fake sweetener is used in more than 6,000 products and it's eaten by more than 200 million people around the world.[1] And while it's classified by the US Food and Drug Administration (FDA) as a "general purpose sweetener" I prefer to call it "bad news."

Aspartame sounds fine and dandy—until you start looking at its sordid past and the results of a very concerning recent study. Researchers at Brigham and Women's Hospital and Harvard Medical School conducted this recent test. It looked at the relationship between drinking regular and diet soft drinks and risks of lymphoma and leukemia in more than 77,000 women and 47,000 men over 22-years. Researchers found that drinking more than one serving of diet soda a day was associated in certain groups with increased risk of developing leukemia, multiple myeloma, and non-Hodgkin's lymphomas compared with participants who do not drink as much diet soda.[2] More specifically it found that greater intake of diet soda was associated with:

- higher leukemia risk in men and women (pooled analysis)

- higher multiple myeloma risk (in men only)

- higher risk non-Hodgkin's lymphoma risk (in men only)

The type of analysis done in this study doesn't *prove* by itself that aspartame causes cancer. But it's another great reason to avoid the sweetener. Or at least, use it sparingly. Aspartame eventually breaks down into formaldehyde a chemical that can cause cancer. The main source of this potential poison is diet soda.

Your brain on aspartame

Aspartame is made of two amino acids, aspartic acid and phenylalanine *combined* with a methyl ester group. Now you don't need to remember all those 20 cent words. Instead, just remember that according to some reports aspartame may wreak havoc on your brain and nervous system. Some critics of the sweetener believe that it acts as an excitotoxin—a chemical substance that damages neurons by stimulating excess activity. It's also been widely reported that the Food and Drug Administration (FDA) has received more than 10,000 complaints about aspartame. These complaints included headaches, dizziness, and even seizures.

Don't settle for sucralose

Sucralose, known by the retail name Splenda, is a common artificial sweetener in the US. No long-term human studies have been conducted on Splenda. And the studies done on animals aren't reassuring. They reveal links to reduced thymus growth rate…enlargement of the liver and kidneys…decreased packed cell volume…and increased risk of cataracts. Admittedly, the amount of sucralose fed to the study animals was very high—yet there's still a great need for clinical studies on humans.

Saccharin side effects?

Saccharin, sold as Sweet'N Low and Necta Sweet, has been a controversial artificial sweetener since its introduction in the early 1900s. Some users report reactions to saccharin, including itching, hives, headache, and diarrhea. A study done in the late 1970s showed that high doses can cause bladder cancer in male rats. Based on those findings saccharin was banned in Canada (but they're considering lifting the ban). In 1977, Congress required warning labels for products containing saccharin, although this requirement has since been repealed.

Beware: Artificial sweeteners could have bitter consequences for your health

I have been warning you about the dangers of artificially sweetened beverages for years. Now it appears that those in conventional circles are finally taking notice.

In a new, as yet unpublished, Italian study, rodents given sucralose (better known as the brand name Splenda) had a higher risk of leukemia. The higher the dose of the artificial sweetener, the higher the risk was.

The findings are troubling, to say the least. In fact, the nonprofit food safety watchdog group, Center for Science in the Public Interest, reacted to the news with the decision to downgrade sucralose's rating from "safe" to the "caution" category in its newest guide to food additives.[1] In the past, sucralose has already been linked with belly problems including bloating, nausea, and gas, and some users have even complained of dizzy spells and memory loss.

But it's not just sucralose that we need to be concerned about… not by a long shot. More troubling research regarding all artificial sweeteners has been surfacing. Dr. Swithers, a professor of behavioral neuroscience at Purdue University recently published a scathing new review based on a growing pile of published studies over the last forty years. The professor warned that users of sugar substitutes may, "…be at increased risk of excessive weight gain, metabolic syndrome, type 2 diabetes, and cardiovascular disease."[2]

You see, fake sugar essentially tricks your body into thinking you're the eating the real calories normally associated with sweet tastes. But of course there are no calories with artificial sweeteners so your body stops releasing the hormones that tell you to stop eating. And, to make matters worse the dopamine that your body typically releases to give you a feeling of satisfaction when you eat something sweet never gets triggered.

In other words, when you gulp down that diet soda you never get the proper "stop" signal. As a result you end up eating more… and often that more is the junk food that you should be avoiding.

So, ironically, the research is finding that although many people turn to diet soda and other foods sweetened with fake sugar to manage weight, heart, and blood sugar issues those artificially sweetened foods are actually putting them at a higher risk. For example, earlier this year a French study found that women who drink large amounts of diet soda may be at an increased risk for type 2 diabetes.[3]

The bottom line is artificial sweeteners may monkey with blood sugar, alter your brain chemistry, and even put you at a higher risk for cancer. My advice is to avoid all of them including Acesulfame, Aspartame, Neotame, Saccharin, and Sucralose. Instead try safe natural sweeteners such as honey, Stevia, Erythritol, and Lo Han.

Article Citations:

1. CSPI Downgrades Splenda From "Safe" to "Caution" http://cspinet.org/new/201306121.html
2. 'Caution' Warranted if Consuming Artificial Sweeteners. Accessed online August 8, 2013 at http://www.medscape.com/viewarticle/807615
3. Fagherazzi, G. et al. Consumption of artificially and sugar-sweetened beverages and incident type 2 diabetes in the Etude Epidémiologique auprès des femmes de la Mutuelle Générale de l'Education Nationale–European Prospective Investigation into Cancer and Nutrition cohort. Am J Clin Nutr. March 2013 ajcn.

Stevia is safe and sweet

Americans have been tricked to believe that artificial sweeteners pose no risk. Here's the truth: In susceptible people, artificial sweeteners may be associated with variety of health problems, from weight gain to headaches to mood changes to possibly cancer. Why take unnecessary risks? There are all-natural alternatives that can satisfy the pickiest sweet tooth, without adding unwanted calories.

Stevia rebaudiana (stevia) has been a popular natural sweetener in the US health food industry for the past 17 years. The plant grows in the rain forests of Brazil and Paraguay, and in Asia. Stevia is up to 300 times sweeter than table sugar and has almost no calories. I have found it has no detrimental effects on blood sugar readings.

In studies, stevia lowered blood pressure in people with mild hypertension and reduced blood glucose levels in patients with type-2 diabetes. Also, an extract from stevia leaves contains antioxidant polyphenol flavonoids which protect against DNA damage, according to a study published in *the Journal of Agricultural and Food Chemistry*.[3]

Stevia is available in liquid, powder, and tablet form. To sweeten an eight-ounce beverage, such as coffee, tea, or lemonade, you generally need to use only one tablet, a pinch of the powder, or three to five drops of the liquid. Follow directions on the label.

You can bake with stevia, substituting one teaspoon of powder or liquid extract for each cup of sugar. Stevia can have a bitter aftertaste, depending on the brand and amount used. Fortunately recent stevia extracts have less of the bitter aftertaste that was once a problem. Even soda pop conglomerates Pepsi and Coca Cola are introducing products sweetened with stevia.

The xylitol option

Xylitol is a white substance that looks and tastes like sugar. You find the natural sweetener in fruits, vegetables, and the bark of some trees. The human body also produces xylitol naturally while breaking down other food sources. In the 1960s it was approved as a food additive by both the World Health Organization and the FDA. Xylitol has 40 to 50 percent fewer calories than sugar. It has no detrimental effects on blood sugar levels and is safe for people with diabetes.

Xylitol has another surprising benefit. The sweetener reduces the formation of cavity-causing plaque. It does this by preventing bacteria from adhering to the mucous membranes of the mouth and sinus and helps to build tooth enamel. Xylitol is used in sugar-free chewing gums, mouthwashes, and toothpastes—products I buy for my own family.

This natural sweetener works very well for beverages. However, xylitol should not be used for baking breads or other foods that contain yeast. In some people, xylitol can trigger diarrhea. To avoid this, start with a small amount and let your digestive tract adjust to it gradually. Xylitol is available in powder form. One popular product is Xylosweet.

The zero calorie fruit extract

Lo han kuo (also spelled luo han guo) is the fruit of *Momordica grossvenori* plant, a member of the cucumber family that grows in southern China. For several centuries, the fruit has been used by practitioners of Chinese medicine to treat dry coughs, sore throats, skin conditions, digestive problems, and to calm the nervous system. People make tea, juice, soup, candy and cake from the dried fruits.

It contains no sugar or calories, and it's safe for people with diabetes and hypoglycemia (low blood sugar). It doesn't lose its sweetness when heated, so it can be used in baking and cooking. The FDA has approved lo han kuo as a "generally regarded as safe" (GRAS) food ingredient. There's no known toxicity associated with this fruit extract. Lo han kuo products I find have a taste similar to maple syrup and leave no aftertaste.

One product that's been popular with my patients is Lo Han Sweet made by the company Jarrow. It's a combination of Lo Han and Xylitol. It can be found online and in health food stores.

Sources:

1. Calorie Control Council website Aspartame Information Center. Accessed November 25, 2012 at www.aspartame.org.

2. Schernhammer ES, Bertrand KA, Birmann BM, Sampson L, Willett WC, Feskanich D. Consumption of artificial sweetener–and sugar-containing soda and risk of lymphoma and leukemia in men and women. American Journal of Clinical Nutrition 2012;96:1419–28.

3. S. Ghanta, el al., Oxidative DNA damage preventive activity and antioxidant potential of Stevia rebaudiana (Bertoni) Bertoni, a natural sweetener. The Journal of Agricultural and Food Chemistry(2007)

#3: Sugary Drinks Can Boost Endometrial Cancer Risk

Sugar boosts cancer risk in women

I don't think anyone should be drinking sugary drinks at all — because even in moderation, soda and other soft drinks can do real damage to men, women and children alike.

But ladies, today I want to focus on you — because new research finds that women who drink the sweet stuff have a much higher risk of endometrial cancer.

Sugar of course causes blood sugar levels to spike and alters the body's insulin response. What makes a soda habit in particular so damaging is that it causes those sugar levels to spike and plunge quickly.

When it happens too often, you get insulin resistance and diabetes.

But even if you don't suffer from diabetes, changes to insulin and insulin growth factor proteins can lead to cancer — including estrogen-dependent endometrial cancer.

That's why any sugary drinks at all will cause your risk of this form of cancer to rise. The risk gets higher with every sip — and if you drink soda regularly, your risk of this disease will jump by nearly 80 percent, according to the study of 23,039 postmenopausal women tracked for up to 25 years.

Along with sugary drinks, the study also finds some other risk factors for this cancer — including a few we already know about: age, obesity, diabetes and early puberty or late menopause.

You don't have any control over your age or when menopause strikes. But you do have control over your weight and you can take steps to avoid diabetes — and avoiding soda will help you to do both at the same time.

Switch to water or seltzer instead. If you want a little flavor, infuse some fruit into it. And if you want a drink that will cut your risk of disease, including several types of cancer, try some tea.

#4: Cellphone Use Linked to Brain Cancer

For years, you've heard that cellphones are safe. Sure, there have been studies that have shown otherwise — but the moment they've come out, the talking heads have rushed to dismiss them.

Now, new research again links cellphones to brain tumors. And again, you wouldn't know it from much of the media coverage.

First, the part you're missing: Regular cellphone users — people who use them just 15 hours a month, or 30 minutes a day — have between double and triple the risk of a brain tumor over five years, according to the study in *British Occupational and Environmental Medicine*.

But even the study itself seems to be hiding this conclusion, because by the researchers' definition, "regular" cellphone users had no higher risk of a tumor at all.

How'd they get away with that? It's all in the definitions.

They defined a "regular" cellphone user as someone who's on the device just once a week, and those who used the cellphones for 15 hours a month were considered "heavy" users.

And by those definitions, only "heavy" users faced the higher tumor risk.

Pretty tricky, huh?

I don't know many people who pony up money for voice and data plans just to use the thing once a week, so I think it's pretty safe to say that 15 hours a month is practically nothing for many people.

Some of my kids' friends seem to be on them 15 hours a day!

Even many adults have gotten rid of their landlines and use only cellphones now — and combined with unlimited voice plans, they're on them all the time and certainly use them for 15 hours a month or more.

But you don't have to get rid of your cell completely. Just be smart about how you use it — and I've got three simple tips that can do just that for you.

First, never hold a cellphone to your head. The increased risk is almost certainly caused by the radiation emitted from the phone — a type of radiation similar to what's emitted by microwaves, which is a known carcinogen.

When you hold a phone against your ear, you're aiming that radiation right at your brain.

Cellphone makers say the answer is to hold the phone a couple of inches from your ear instead of right up against it, but good luck trying to hear your callers that way.

Instead, get a set of headphones with a built-in microphone. Many phones, especially smartphones, come with them — and most people don't use them. Use them, or invest in a better pair.

You'll hear your callers better, they'll hear you better and you'll minimize the risk to your brain.

If you're in a quiet room, you can even use the speakerphone function.

Second, don't keep the phone in a pocket or on your hip, or anywhere else on your body, as emerging evidence shows they can harm fertility and even cause bone loss when they're attached to you all day long.

And finally, I would also suggest not getting rid of your landline just yet. Use it at home instead of your cell, and not just for health reasons.

In the event of an emergency such as a natural disaster, landlines are much more likely to remain functional than cellphones.

#5: Mouthwash Linked to Oral Cancer Symptoms

Why you shouldn't use mouthwash

It's another "good" habit that's actually bad for you — and millions of people do it two or three times a day or more.

It's a quick swish with some mouthwash. It's supposed to kill germs, freshen your breath and protect your teeth. That's what it says on the label anyway, and you certainly feel fresher and smell better after that rinse.

But new research confirms it's also doing something else: It could be causing oral cancer symptoms.

People who use mouthwash — especially people who use it three times a day or more — have a higher risk of oral cancers symptoms, new research confirms. So do people who don't take care of their mouths at all.

In other words, a mouthwash habit could be about as bad for you as poor dental hygiene, at least when it comes to your cancer risk.

While some people are surprised by the new study, I'm not. Alcohol is a known carcinogen, and when you let it circulate in the delicate tissues of the mouth several times a day, of course it's going to do some damage.

That's why heavy drinkers and alcoholics have a higher risk of oral cancers (among other problems).

Smoking can also boost the odds, and smokers who use mouthwash have the biggest oral cancer risk of all.

That's a pretty common combination, too, since many smokers are always using mouthwash.

They're trying to mask the nasty smell of nicotine breath. It doesn't really work — you can still smell a smoker a mile away — but it does do something else: alcohol and nicotine, when combined, form a highly cancerous compound called acetaldehyde.

It's so dangerous that a 2009 study found that smokers who use mouthwash have 9 times the cancer risk.

If you need to freshen up, use an all-natural alcohol-free rinse instead.

But if you're just looking to care for your mouth, you don't need any type of mouthwash or rinse at all. All you need is some floss and a quality all-natural (and fluoride-free) toothpaste.

Brush and floss after meals, and you'll have the cleanest mouth in town.